# MASTER YOUR MIND MASTER YOUR MOOD

# MASTER YOUR MIND MASTER YOUR MOOD

## Navigate your way to success and happiness

**Dr Steven Thomas**

Distributed by SwordWorks Books, UK

ISBN 978-1-906512-35-4

# FOREWORD

Mood related illnesses have become increasingly prevalent in modern Western society. So much so that there is, or at least there seems to be, almost an epidemic of depression, anxiety and similar difficulties across the whole spectrum of society. There are a number of approaches to these kinds of problems, ranging from traditional psychiatric treatment to somewhat extreme and often untried methods such as the more mystical aspects coming out of the Asian continent.

We firmly believe that there is no single route to an effective cure and relief of symptoms of depression and mood related illness. Instead, it is almost beyond doubt that a more holistic approach is required. To this end we are offering the sufferer a whole range of tools, most requiring some kind of interaction and feedback along the way that in combination will certainly mitigate the worst aspects of depressive illness and at best could cure completely the symptoms in many patients.

We urge you to read through this book in its entirety and to experiment with the tools and techniques you find there. Choose the ones that suit you, the ones that work for you, and work with them to improve your health. Most importantly, what is required from you is action. This is a self-help programme, there is no one to tell you when to start and when to stop and to make certain that you follow any kind of an orderly regime of treatment.

The amount of progress you make is entirely up to you. This is an exciting prospect; you should see it as a tremendous empowerment after a period when you will undoubtedly have been feeling disempowered and disabled by your symptoms. Take the chance and go for it, even if you only do a little you cannot fail. If you use the book to its fullest extent the likelihood of success is very high indeed.

We wish you good health and good mood.


Dr Steven Thomas

# CONTENTS

# INTRODUCTION

# INTRODUCTION

What do we mean by mood? Different people may well have different interpretations. However, most would take and assume mood to be an emotional state either simple or more complex, at the extreme end of which it becomes depression, and the extreme end of depression is of course a severe clinical depression. It would however, be less than helpful to label low mood per se as depression. Of course, in more severe cases it can be used as a suitable label where an accurate diagnosis is required to help the patient to recover from their symptoms. Suffice to say that when we talk about mood we are talking about the whole range of negative emotions ranging from being slightly "fed up" to severe clinical depression.

Of course mood can also be positive, when people feel that their lives are balanced, they are happy and optimistic and looking forward to the future. This is the aim of this book, to take you to this positive mood level. It is by no means an overnight task. However it should be an enjoyable task, one in which you will begin to feel the benefits from the very start sufficiently to keep you going on the programme until you find that your life really has changed for the better.

The various therapies for curing low mood will tend to be used in different combinations for different people. Everyone is different, people exhibit different temperaments, personality traits and in some cases certain neuroses and anxieties. Some people are long-term sufferers, other people's suffering is intermittent or site click, other people have only recently begun to feel the negative experience of low mood. So there are a wide variety of conditions and people, only you can make the final decision as to what works are you and then continued to use it.

The diagnostic and statistical manual of mental disorders defines depression as feelings of sadness, helplessness and hopelessness. You may just feel sad but it could be nonetheless one and the same thing. Or not. We offer in this book a range of methods of gauging whether or not your low mood is sufficient to be classed as depressive. You can then go further to confirm your assessment by consulting a professional therapist. The therapist may recommend treatment, and from there you can go on to make decisions about your treatment.

We do not offer an alternative to treatment. That would be impossible, given the incredibly diverse numbers of people types, and illness types. Only a therapist can do that. What we can offer is a range of therapies that will certainly improve your symptoms, either in conjunction with the prescribed therapies or, subject to professional approval, as a separate, standalone set of treatments.

## INTRODUCTION

We cannot advise individuals about the taking of prescribed medication. Obviously it can and does work very well in a great number of situations. Equally, where people have stopped taking their medication early, they have suffered very badly. Then again, there are many recorded cases of where prescribed medication has done more harm than good. It is complicated, the only way forward is to discuss it with your therapist and reach a decision with their assistance and agreement.

Remember, no matter how difficult and how complicated your illness may seem, you have taken that important first step by recognising it and beginning to deal with it.

This part of the book introduces some of the key concepts such as the Mind Compass and helps you to understand some of the underlying causes of various moods. Several cases are examined and at the end of the chapter you will find a list of useful exercises to carry out to help reinforce your learning.

# CHAPTER 1: MIND COMPASS

# CHAPTER 1: MIND COMPASS

*I am a contradictory mess but I see it as my prerogative to change
my mood like the weather.*

*Shirley Manson*

We need to look at the whole question of what governs both your physical and your mental well-being. It is almost certainly the case that no single symptom will result in the complexities reported by patients seeking help for their emotional challenges and difficulties. It is of course the case that no two people are exactly alike. However, we have identified a fairly simple diagram which will assist you in understanding the various threads that come together to underline the emotional health of any particular person. Think of the points of the compass, north, south, east and west. In a similar way we have devised a four point model to illustrate the complex relationships that together form a person's mental health.

We will call this our 'mood compass'.

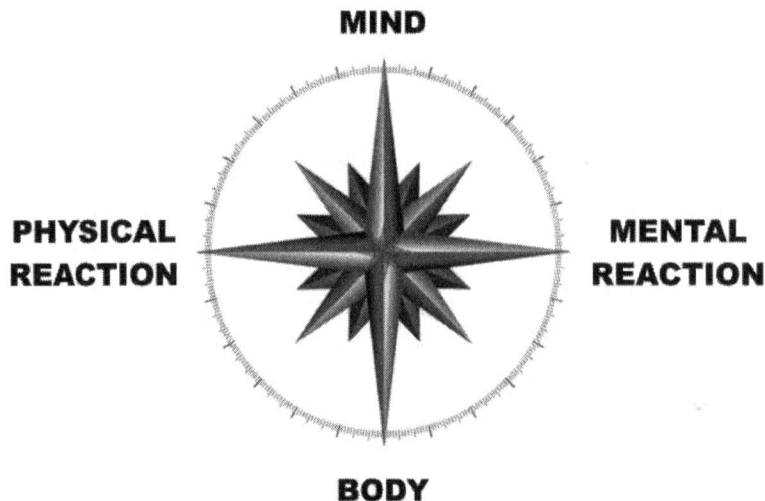

- Instead of North, think of the mind. The mind is that complex hub of physical and emotional influences. A very common characteristic of the mind that causes people to seek help from therapists is low self esteem.

- For South, we need to look at the model of the physical body, which in adversity will display such symptoms as chronic illness, acute illness, allergies and a range of symptoms ranging from a cut finger to severe heart problems.

- To the West of our compass style diagram we have identified physical reactions to a range of stimuli. These could be headaches, aches and pains, stiffness and soreness and occasionally more severe difficulties such as ME.

- Lastly to the East of our compass we can look at mental reactions to stimuli. These reactions are the kinds of things that will result in changes of mood. In the case of people seeking therapy these changes of mood will almost certainly be very severe indeed, at least in so far as the patient is concerned.

It is important to consider, and we hope to demonstrate this in the following case studies, that no single symptom is likely to occur independently. Rather that the person seeking help needs to have their symptoms examined using the four points of the mood compass. For it is indeed the case that a symptom related to one point of the mood compass will certainly be part of a wider set of issues related to all points of the mood compass. As you will see from the actual case studies, the person suffering from low self esteem may well display physical symptoms of such things as aches and pains, as well as a range of emotional or mental reactions such as mood changes, which can often be very sudden. Let's take a look at some cases that illustrate this point more adequately.

## CASE STUDY A

A counsellor was contacted by a middle-aged man named Edward. This man was very concerned with his wife Jane who was sixty years old. Jane's recent behaviour had caused Edward to be very worried about her. The evening before he

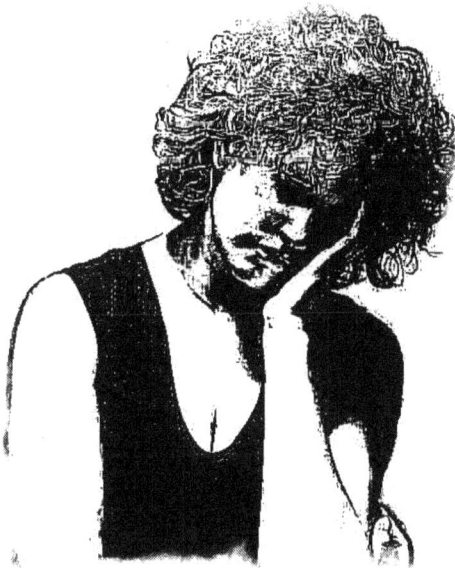

had watched a television documentary on the growing problem of depression and how its treatment was difficult and occasionally very controversial. For several weeks Edward's wife Jane had apparently been suffering from fairly severe insomnia. She seemed to find it difficult to get to sleep at night and even when she did get to sleep she tended to frequently wake up and just read a book or wander around the house doing odd jobs. Normally not a problem, but at three and five o'clock in the morning this was obviously unusual behaviour, especially in that previously she had kept fairly routine hours of sleep. Perhaps unsurprisingly, as a result of this interrupted sleeping pattern, Jane said that she was constantly tired throughout the day, and did not feel able to carry on with her normal activities. For most of her life she had been a keen and enthusiastic ballroom dancer, winning several medals when she was younger. Jane had kept up her dancing in later life and was part of a team of dance enthusiasts who went around old people's homes showing the residents how to use gentle dance movements and activity. The dancers were encouraging general fitness and staving off the degenerative physical and mental processes of old age. From being an enthusiastic and dynamic member of the team she had almost completely lost interest in this activity and was generally unwilling to participate further when asked.

It was the final symptom of constant irritability towards Edward that had caused him to consider that Jane may be suffering from depression. Following the television documentary he contacted the counsellor and persuaded Jane to make a visit. When Jane went into the counsellor's office she made it clear at the outset that quite simply she was just "getting older". She didn't need any kind of help and indeed if therapy was needed that time should not be wasted on her but given to the old folk in the home is that until recently she had been assisting with dance centred therapy.

In fact this is by no means an unusual reaction in people who are suffering from these kinds of symptoms of insomnia, irritability and lack of energy and enthusiasm for the normal day-to-day activities. They can see that other people around them may need help. In Jane's case the senior citizens in the old people's homes that she had been visiting, but not herself. In this case as in most others, the therapist needs to use the four compass style diagram as a basis of assessment of that particular person's difficulties. The therapist asked Edward to join him and Jane in the consulting room. Edward was the conventional picture of a middle-aged, middle-class man. Aged sixty four years old, smartly dressed in a dark suit with a shirt and tie, clean-shaven, polished shoes and a neat haircut.

Jane presented a slight contrast, in that although of a similar age and social class to her husband, she was in fact slightly unkempt compared to him. Her hair clearly had not been cut for some time and was slightly unkempt, her eyes looked dull and as with most insomniacs she had the dark circles of sleeplessness around them. She remonstrated again that her problems were of little consequence and in fact were just a symptom of growing older. She stated, quite firmly, that this visit would be a total waste of time, but in any case as they were here they should "just get it over with" and then the therapist could move on to more deserving cases. It was encouraging to note that despite her obvious difficulties her prime concern was with others rather than herself.

## SYMPTOMS

The therapist managed to get Jane to respond to his questions, nonetheless, and eventually an emerging picture began to appear. Jane had worked for most of her life as a translator for a local multinational company. She had brought up two children and was proud of the fact that the efforts of her husband and herself had resulted in both children were going to university and taking up successful careers, one in law and the other as a chemical engineer. Both her and her husband had earned good salaries and had been able to give their family a balanced and rewarding lifestyle as a result.

Eight months previously Edward had suffered a mild heart attack requiring a stay in hospital. Fortunately the heart attack was not symptomatic of a more serious heart problem, rather it served as an early warning for Edward to modify his lifestyle, changing his diet and taking more exercise to prevent a further and more serious heart problem occurring. Since then, Edward had been clear of any further heart difficulties and in fact his general health was showing a marked and continuing improvement. Edward's illness had shocked Jane into realising how potentially close she had come to losing her husband of thirty eight years.

Shortly after Edward came out of hospital one of Jane's companions in her dance group was diagnosed with a brain tumour. It appeared that she could be treated by a mild operation to remove the tumour which was not in a life-threatening place. However, when she came out of hospital she never really recovered from the operation. It seems that the condition was more serious than had at first been diagnosed and four months ago this person died. Jane had been particularly close to this person and following on from her husband's illness the death seemed to affect her very deeply. On the one hand husband had been treated and recovered very well, yet her friend whose diagnosis seemed to be similarly optimistic had not survived.

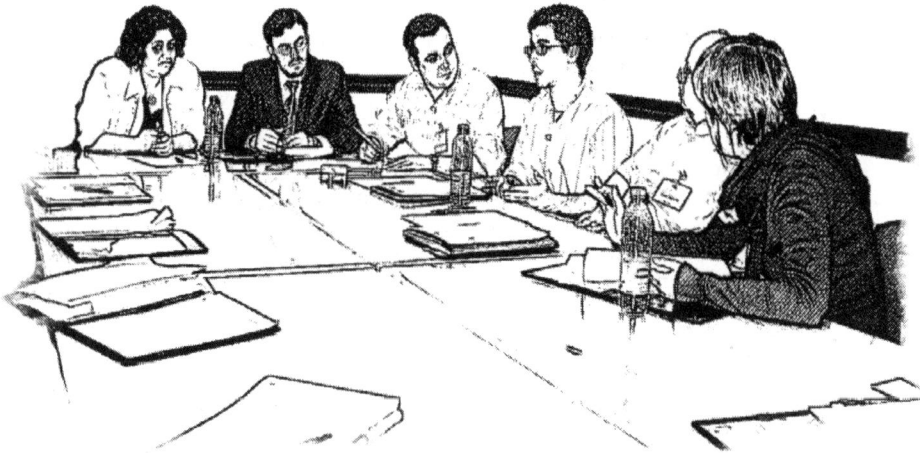

She dwells endlessly on the reasons for the death of her friend and the survival of her husband. Surely if her husband had survived, should not her friend have survived a diagnosis that was in essence no more life-threatening than his. Should she be more concerned about her husband's future prospects for survival? Was he about to die? Had her friend died as a result of some kind of medical mistake or misdiagnosis? These questions preoccupied endlessly. She spent more and more time obsessing about her husband's care and welfare, worrying that at any time he could be struck down and die. She no longer went to her dance group and essentially her life was a succession of morbid thoughts as she tottered around the house worrying about her husband's prospects in the future. At the same time her thoughts caused her to be increasingly susceptible to insomnia, which in itself caused her to be increasingly irritable during the day. As an active person previously she had now stopped all forms of exercise, especially the practice of dance which had been an important factor in her mental and physical well-being of the whole of her life. This resulted in her becoming less fit and even more irritable as she was unable to experience the sheer joy and release of the exercise and movement she loved.

## ANALYSIS

Using the four-point mind compass it was possible to look at Jane's difficulties and understand them in a relatively straightforward way. In this way the four points could each be examined in isolation and then to see how they interacted with each other, coming together to form those things that were such a debilitating effect on her life.

- her mind was convinced that she was growing old and that her lack of interest in dance and insomnia was a natural result of this ageing process

- her mental reaction was one of increasing irritability

- her physical reaction was to feel less fit as a result of her difficulties and lack of normal exercise routine

- her body reaction was in insomnia, which itself caused her to suffer the previous three difficulties in increasing amounts

We were able to explain to Jane all of these things so that she could understand them. Whilst it may be difficult to take in the whole process of debilitation in one go, once the four points can be dealt with one by one, it becomes clear that they are quite able to react with each other. This may be in such a way that makes it difficult, if not impossible, for the person concerned to find their way out of the problem. In this particular case Jane was able to completely recover from the problems she was experiencing. She could see how the problems with her husband and with her friend had combined to affect her so deeply, and how the various threads of her life had interacted with each other in such a way as to cause her such difficulties.

We were able to help her to deal with these problems one by one, until eventually she was completely free of them and able to understand how and why they had occurred. She made a complete recovery and is once again helping her senior citizens to enjoy their dance classes. She is sleeping well and her married life is once again happy and fulfilled.

## CASE STUDY B

Our second case study concerns a lady we shall name Susan. Susan was suffering from extremely low self esteem and had recently divorced. Apparently her marriage was very traumatic and yet the divorce had not given her the relief she had hoped for and expected. Susan was a lecturer at a college of further education. She had on three occasions taken extended leave of absence, citing sickness. On two of these occasions she had travelled a long distance away to stay with a friend in France (Susan's home and place of work was in London). Her friend had tried to persuade her, with extreme difficulty, to return to England

and her place of work. Susan's attitude was that quite simply everything in London, her home, her work, her broken marriage, her social life, meant nothing at all and had only brought her misery. The only solution she could think of was literally to run away, leaving it all behind and start again. She felt severely depressed.

It appeared that Susan's difficulties had come to a head when her work at the college, which until now had involved principally research, had now changed. She had been assigned to teach a number of classes in front of large numbers of students, possibly as many as a hundred, in the college lecture theatre. The prospect of standing in front of and lecturing so many people was causing her to feel panicky, to the extent that the old feeling of "running away" was beginning to resurface. She literally did not know how to cope, either with her professional life or indeed any part of her life away from her work. She reported that she felt as if she was forever trying to walk through treacle, as if her every movement was much slower than normal. She also reported that physical exercise, even the simple act of walking was causing her a degree of aching in her limbs.

We managed to persuade Susan to discuss her difficulties. She arrived in the consulting room looking considerably older than her thirty three years. She was dressed more like a middle-aged housewife than a college lecturer. She was in cheap ill fitting clothes, a hairstyle that looked as if she had cut and styled it herself without any real ability. She was about three stones overweight and sadly her clothes had been bought at a time before she put on the excess weight and so they were stretched very tight around her.

After a series of discussions we established that her symptoms correlated very strongly with the four-point mind compass.

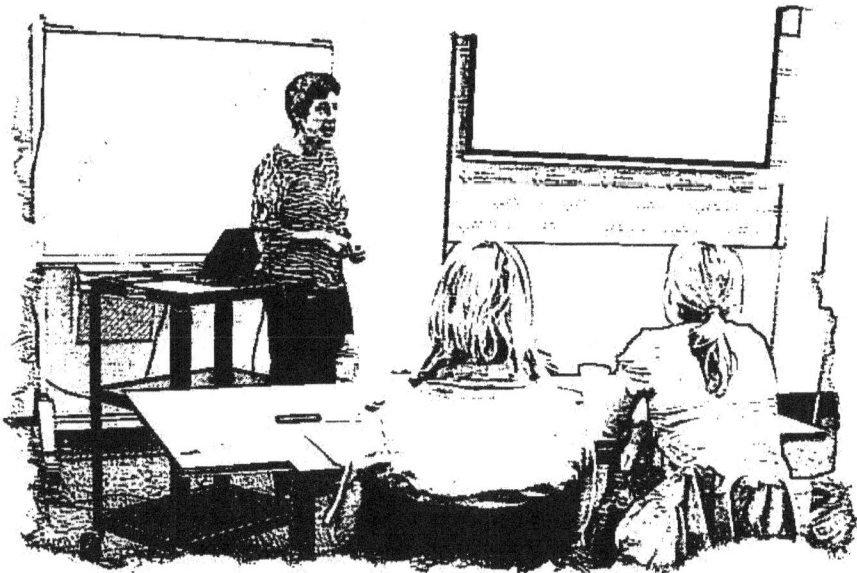

## SYMPTOMS

The northerly symptom, that of mind, was very open and evident. She felt an almost total lack of self esteem. As a person she felt she could bring nothing at all to any kind of relationship. She was of no use to her students in the college and her marriage had failed for reasons that must have been to do with her lack of positive input. Her lack of esteem seemed to be something she wore like a badge in her ill fitting clothes, almost as if she was trying to show the world how little she was worth.

- The southerly symptom, that of bodily symptoms, was clearly evident for everyone to see. This formerly smart and attractive young woman, maintaining a successful vocation as a college lecturer, had become very overweight. In her ill fitting clothes she seemed to be either unable or unprepared to do anything about correcting her obvious weight problem.

- Looking towards the east of our mind compass, we examine the symptoms of physical reaction in this person's difficulties. The mental pain of her low self esteem with the increasing physical difficulty of keeping mobile in the face of the unaccustomed increase in weight was causing a healthy young woman, formerly with no obvious health problems or experience of chronic pain, to experience an increasing degree of aches and pains when carrying out the most demanding functions ie walking short distances.

- In the west of our mind compass we examine mental reactions to the person's difficulties. In this particular case the combination of factors had brought about the onset of panic attacks when Susan was faced with the prospect of dealing with a lecture room filled with people.

During the second session of discussions with Susan we established that as a child she felt that she was being physically abused by her father. It seemed that the onset of low self-esteem started at this point. She had never discussed this abuse with any other person. Instead it seemed to be lurking in the background of her mind to surface when other pressures closed in around her. It seemed that the panic attacks were an irregular feature of her life, appearing at times of stress such as during the period of her divorce and at the point of her being assigned to normal teaching duties. The attacks took the form of the onset of severe headache together with a paralysis like state of the mind, so that she felt frozen, unable to go in any direction or make any definite decisions. There was also the overwhelming compulsion to run away completely from what she perceived as the source of her misery.

## ANALYSIS

There seems to be no single reason why Susan should have suffered these attacks. Rather it seemed that a combination of factors had built on each other, building towards the full-blown set of symptoms which we see on the mind compass, to the point where they upset her life completely and caused such misery to her. After further discussions we were able to identify the source of the panic attacks with stages of her life that followed degrees of change. The underlying problem of low self esteem was always a trap into which she would fall when other factors combined to upset the stability of her life, such as the divorce and the change in working practice from research to teaching a class.

Susan reported that during the panic attacks she suffered symptoms such as the paralysis or numbness of her brain, making it very difficult to think of the way forward. She could feel her heart beating so much that she felt that anyone standing close would be able to hear the thump thump of its beat. Her breathing occasionally became difficult, especially when the beating of her heart seems to palpitate making it difficult for her to breathe in and out normally.

Although Susan initially was reporting depression, or at least feelings of depression, you can see that it quickly became obvious to us that there were a number of factors that were contributing towards her problem. We were able to explain each stage of the problems to her, using the four-point mind compass model. Once her problems were separated so that she could examine them and deal with them one by one, rather than as a huge black and frightening mass, she was able to deal with those things that were causing her so much pain. She once more began to eat properly and started to lose some of the excess weight she had acquired. She had managed to get the problems of abuse as a child into the open and discuss them with a third party, so that she could realise that she was in no way responsible. She was just a victim that needed to be helped over this painful part of her past. With the emotional relief of getting over this hurdle of discussing this painful subject, together with reverting to a healthier diet, Susan was able to once again enjoy being more physically active. This again helped her physical and mental self image and increased her store of confidence to overcome the panic attacks that seemed to leading her life out of control.

Today, Susan is a successful teacher, once again smart and attractive, and able to enjoy the fruits of the life she has worked so hard to achieve.

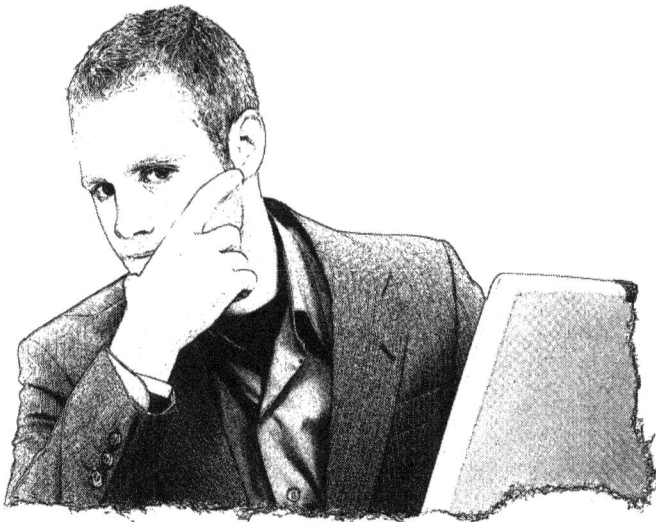

## CASE STUDY C

Let's look at one more example of a patient who we have been able to help. We will call this man Tony. He is aged fifty five and has acknowledged that he is addicted to cocaine. Indeed he has stated that his need for cocaine is related to his working life, which involves a very high flying senior management post in a city of London brokerage house. Tony arrived at our office looking every inch the successful business professional. The suit was quite definitely Armani or Versace, perhaps something similar or even more expensive. His shoes looked handmade by one of the small and exclusive London bootmakers and had that sheen of expensive and well cared for leather. His hair was equally well groomed and immaculate and he was clean shaven. Perhaps the only indication that there was a problem was in his face, which looked fit and tanned. Only as he moved closer could an observer see that the tan looked very much the product of a tanning studio and behind it there was a face that looked fairly patchy and strained.

He felt the need to take cocaine many years previously when he was an up and coming broker. For many years he worked long hours under the kind of intense pressure that perhaps most people would be unable to tolerate. He was introduced by a colleague to cocaine. From initial dismay and disgust at the thought of taking an illegal drug he found that after taking cocaine his performance at work, which had recently started to decline, was drastically improved, so much so that he was promoted. Lately the reverse has been true and he found that, not only did taking cocaine do nothing at all to improve his performance, he had in fact become prone to making mistakes that threatened to become severe enough to cost him his job.

## ANALYSIS

Tony had always been something of a driving personality, often described as a "Type A" personality. He had been brought up to believe that if he worked hard, and was extremely careful to make sure that every effort he made was checked and double checked and was literally perfect, he would be successful. He was also taught that the opposite was true, that if he relaxed his guard for one moment and did not control and double check every aspect of his work he would be unsuccessful and would be likely to wind up in the gutter.

The reason for Tony seeking help was that he saw himself as in an impossible situation. He felt that he needed the cocaine to operate at a sufficiently high level to hold down his job, especially in the face of younger people in the company that he always saw as looking enviously at his job and waiting for the day when they could usurp him. At the same time the cocaine was not giving him the initial boost than it used to, so that he was well aware that he was hopelessly addicted and paying huge sums of money from his salary just to maintain the dose. Remembering his parents' warnings and admonitions, he was terrified of losing his job and winding up "in the gutter" as they always told him would be the reward for failure.

He had begun to experience feelings of sickness and frequent severe headaches. His weight had begun to decline and it turned out that his expensive suit had twice been altered to suit his declining body size. He now felt that dealing with the younger members of staff in his company was becoming increasingly impossible, that they were sneering at his declining figure and just waiting for the chance to "stick the knife in" as soon as his guard was dropped. He found it difficult to sleep and frequently woke up in the night terrified that the next day would find him dismissed from his job and on his way "to the gutter".

It was clear to us from the outset that Tony was a very experienced and accomplished professional. He was competent and good at his job but impeded by his terrors of the price of failure, which presumably had been a contributing factor in his decision to start taking cocaine to improve his performance and ward off the risk of this terrible consequence ever happening.

Looking at the mind compass we can see clearly that his state of mind had already been determined by his parents continually undermining his self-confidence by persistently spelling out the terrible consequence of failure. After all, the reality is that many people attempt a career path and find that they are unsuited to it. This is not failure. The average person will merely look for a different and more appropriate career. As a result Tony had started taking cocaine which undermined his physiology whilst at the same time gave a very temporary and artificial boost to his mental functions. This caused him to begin losing weight and suffer the physical reactions that are a consequence of taking the illegal drug cocaine. He tried to counter act this with artificial tanning which was only partially successful. His face, instead of looking like that of a successful executive just returned from the Caribbean, was more of a ghastly caricature. As a result of all of these factors he reacted mentally by experiencing increasing feelings of terror at the thought of other young staff members taking over his job and driving him to the very depths which he had spent his life being terrified of.

Of course it was necessary in the case of Tony to advocate a course of therapy to rid him of his ruinous cocaine habit. Simultaneous with this therapy we were able to demonstrate the four points of the mind compass that had brought him to such a low state. Whilst it may well be necessary to operate on a much higher plane in certain occupations, such as managing city brokerage houses, there are many ways to achieve this higher plane on a permanent and healthy basis. This quite the opposite of the temporary and desperate fix offered by using cocaine.

Eventually Tony was weaned off of cocaine totally and joined a very expensive gymnasium situated in the basement of the city offices where he worked. He found that by living a healthy lifestyle and understanding and dealing with the source of his fears, terrors and other problems he was able to function to the very highest levels of his natural ability. It was this natural ability that had taken him to such a good position in his company in the first place, not an illegal drug habit. Once he realised this, and indeed realised that the very failure that he had been terrified of ever since his childhood was a myth, he was able to regain all of his functions and carry out his work successfully.

## TASKS

At the end of this first chapter there are some tasks for you to carry out so that you get the absolute best out of it:-

1.  Draw a simple mood compass on a sheet of paper as described at the start of the chapter and fill in at each of the four points of the compass those aspects that you feel are causing you difficulties.

2.  Go back through the chapter and on a separate sheet of paper write down those aspects of the three examples given that you feel may apply to you.

3.  Lastly, it will be clear from the foregoing that many existing problems have a history that can go back many years, frequently to childhood. Do you have childhood memories that cause you to feel worried or afraid? On a further sheet of paper write them down.

4.  Now draw a second mind compass and using what you have written for number two and number three, writing the relevant details and compare the completed mind compass to the first mind compass you made. It may well be that the comparison will surprise you, but in any case you can now throw the first mind compass away and use the second mood compass to direct you further on the path to recovery.

*I don't wait for moods. You accomplish nothing if you do that.*
*Your mind must know it has got to get down to work.*

*Pearl S. Buck*

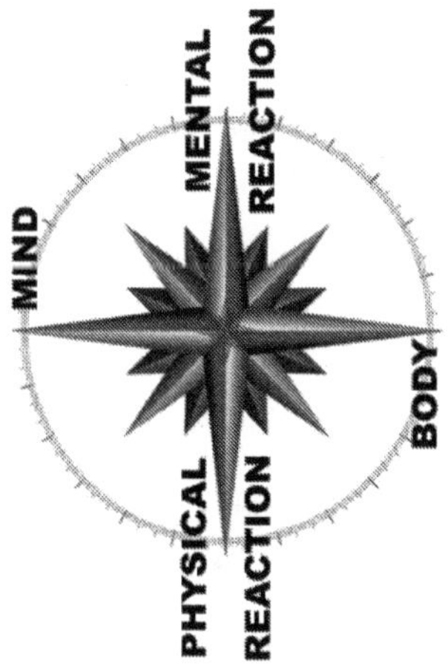
MENTAL
REACTION
MIND
BODY
PHYSICAL
REACTION

This part of the book is about understanding how multiple factors can affect the individual. We will use a selection of example to help you fully understand this part of the book.

# CHAPTER 2: INTERCONNECTION

# CHAPTER 2: INTERCONNECTION

*Time cools, time clarifies; no mood can be maintained quite
unaltered through the course of hours.*

*Thomas Mann*

In chapter 1 we learned that there are a number of factors that contribute to the way we feel about ourselves and the world around us. Everything is interconnected. If you want to feel better about anything or everything in your life it is essential that you understand that you feel the way you do as a result of several different factors. No single factor will have caused the difficulties you are facing, despite the fact that you may well have experienced a very serious setback and blamed everything on that negative event. As an example, let us look at the person who has recently lost her job, has literally been fired totally without warning. That person may well descend into a cycle of anxiety, depression or panic attacks. It would be easy to say " Who wouldn't feel that bad after being fired?" This does not help us to go forward at all. You are asking the wrong question.

The real question should be "How do the majority of people, especially people that are normally happy, contented and fulfilled, react when they suddenly lose their job?". You may well answer that these people would react in a number of different ways. Doubtless you would be right, but consider the number of people that would react by a swift period of feeling miserable and isolated, followed by an intense period of hunting for a new job. Consider the number of people that would be able, after the initial period of adjustment, to say "It was a rotten thing to happen but it could well be the chance for me to find something that I would much prefer to do." There could be a job around the corner that carries a higher salary, or perhaps one that is much more enjoyable and satisfying to do. That would be a normal and sensible way to react to such a difficulty.

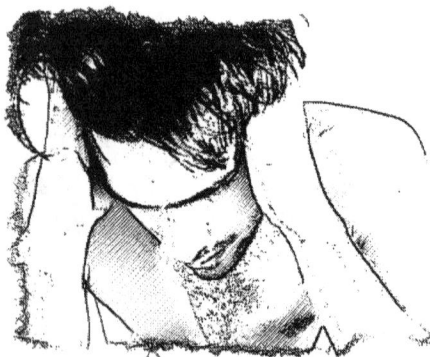

Think back to chapter 1 and the mind compass. If you were to pencil in feelings of anger, of abandonment and isolation, of desperate and uncertain times to come onto your mind compass what are the other points of the compass likely to be completed with? It is unlikely to be a positive, satisfying and helpful outcome. If you have lost your job you need to consider looking at the whole serious of events that led up to it. Subsequently then to work out how you can change them in the way that will be most beneficial to yourself and influence in the best possible way the other factors in your life.

# INTERCONNECTION

Therefore the difference between one person who is going about their lives looking for a new job in a way that is positive and the person who is dwelling on the way they have been treated and how life has little to offer them other than the "stab in the back" is clear. It is a difference purely of perception. It is the way that you actually think of a situation. If you think of yourself as unwanted, possibly unliked, that will certainly lead to an ongoing downward spiral. Almost certainly it will not be true. There are a number of reasons why someone gets sacked from their job and it is extremely rare that they are as personally unliked. You could be unsuitable for the job. Your company may be trying to save money. There could be endless reasons why you have lost your job, equally there could be endless ways you could look at this unfortunate event. It would be self damaging to look at it in any way other than how to put the best possible spin on what has happened. Learn from it and move on, intending to end up in a much better position than before it all happened.

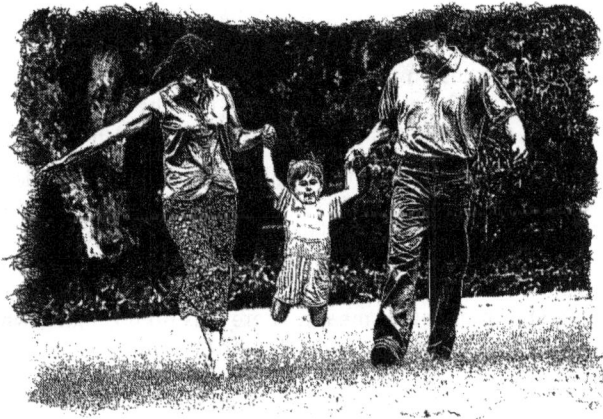

In the case of Jane who was suffering so badly with insomnia, there was a reason for this is that was totally unrelated to her as a person, i.e. she was in no way suffering as a result of old age or infirmity. Yet this was her understanding of her physical and emotional difficulties, that they were all age related. In other words it was not the specific circumstances that were of necessity causing Jane had problems, rather it was her perception of the circumstances. She perceived wrongly that she needed to be excessively concerned over her husband's health, in case his mild heart attack reoccurred in a more severe form, possibly even causing premature death. This would then mean that during the final golden years of her life when she should be enjoying the fruits and benefits of the life that her and her husband had worked so together to achieve, she would be left alone. At the same time the stress that this way of perceiving the problem caused her resulted in a negative effect on her mood, such that she suffered symptoms of insomnia and irritability.

During a time of increased stress brought on by the anxiety of her husband's illness, she suffered a second blow when her good friend died. Again this is a matter of perception. Jane's perception of these events are somehow linked them so that the actual mortality of her friend, though objectively totally isolated from her husband's heart attack, somehow became connected to it. She needed to understand that in fact the two events were completely unrelated. Even more that joining the two events, her husband is a heart attack and her friend's death, resulted not in any kind of resolution or improvement but in a deterioration both of her physical and mental health and in her relationship with her husband, who had become increasingly upset at her irritability.

## EXAMPLE

Here is an interesting story about a well-known violinist that perfectly illustrates this point of perceiving events in ways that will either enhance our lives or seriously crippled them. On November 18th 1995, Itzhak Perlman, the violinist, came on stage to give a concert at Avery Fisher Hall, Lincoln Center, New York City. If you have ever been to a Perlman concert, you know that getting on stage is no small achievement for him. He was stricken with polio as a child and so has braces on both legs and walks with the aid of two crutches. To see him walk across the stage one step at a time, painfully and slowly, is an awesome sight. He walks painfully, yet majestically, until he reaches his chair. Then he sits down slowly, puts his crutches on the floor, undoes the clasps on his legs, tucks one foot back and extends the other foot forward. Then he bends down and picks up the violin, puts it under his chin, nods to the conductor and proceeds to play.

By now, the audience is used to this ritual. They sit quietly while he makes his way across the stage to his chair. They remain reverently silent while he undoes the clasps on his legs. They wait until he is ready to play. But this time, something went wrong. Just as he finished the first few bars, one of the strings on his violin broke. You could hear it snap, it went off like gunfire across the room. There was no mistaking what that sound meant. There was no mistaking what he had to do. People who were there that night thought to themselves he would have to get up, put on the clasps again, pick up the crutches and limp his way off stage to either find another violin or a replacement string.

But he didn't. Instead, he waited a moment, closed his eyes and then signalled the conductor to begin again. The orchestra began and he played from where he had left off. He played with such passion and such power and purity, as they had never heard before. Of course, we all know it is impossible to play a symphonic work with just three strings. I know that, and you know that, but that night Itzhak Perlman refused to know that. You could see him modulating, changing, re-composing the piece in his head. At one point, it sounded like he was de-tuning the strings to get new sounds from them that they had never made before. When he finished, there was an awesome silence in the room and then people rose and cheered. There was an extraordinary outburst of applause throughout the auditorium.

He smiled, wiped the sweat from this brow and raised his bow to quiet the audience. Then he said not boastfully, but in a quiet, pensive, reverent tone "You know, sometimes it is the artist's task to find out how much music you can still make with what you have left.".

Whilst Jane had had nothing like the terrible illness experienced by this violinist, she interpreted her problems in a way that made it far worse. In fact considerably worse in view of the fact that whilst Perlman was severely crippled by his problems her husband had had a very mild illness, a timely warning and was now apparently living a normal healthy and fulfilled life. The difference is all in the perception and the way that you think about a particular problem, difficulty or event. You would do well to consider what problems are troubling you and work out whether or not you can think about them or perceive them in several different ways. Take a sheet of paper, write down one particular problem that you feel distracts from your quality of life and then make a list of several ways in which this problem does affect you.

In Jane's case, she perceived the problem of her husband's mild heart attack as a sign of his mortality and possible early death. She could have, and in fact did eventually see it as a benefit and advantage. Something that gave her warning, that in order for him to live a long and healthy life with her, certain things such as diet and exercise needed to be attended to. Without these changes it could perhaps be the case that he would have had a fatal heart attack at a later time. Yet another perception of this event could be that the changes and modifications in their lifestyles caused them to take a fresh and novel approach to life that until now they had not considered. This could in itself give them an improved quality of life that they had not previously thought of.

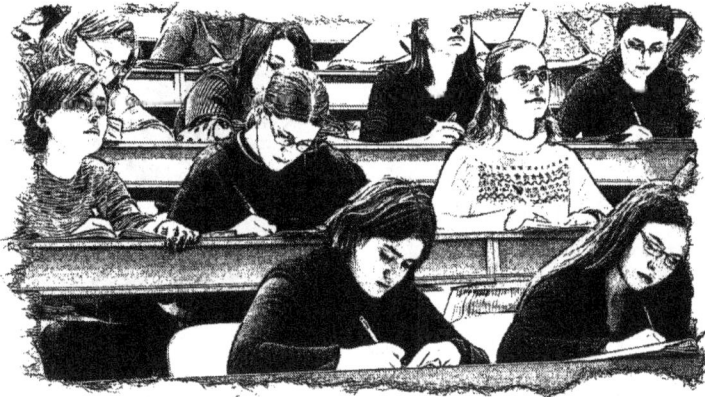

How many more ways could Jane have looked at this mild heart attack? The list is probably endless. As you work on the problem you have written down bear in mind that there will be a number of ways you could perceive it, probably many more than you can think of at the moment. When you have finished put the list to one side. Examine it tomorrow to see if there is anything you could add and in which ways any of these perceptions will make you feel better both about the item on the list and about your life in general.

In Susan's case it is not difficult to understand how her thought process and her perception of life was damaged so badly in the early stages of her life by child abuse. That is one particular case where any kind of different perception is virtually impossible to change the terrible nature of what occurred. However it did, and perhaps the only worthwhile perception of this event would be that it was a long time ago and the only way to throw off the ties to that awful time is to be determined not to be beaten by it. Why should the guilty party cause her to suffer whilst he freely goes about his life, perhaps even abusing other children. The path is clear though sometimes very difficult to resolve because of family ties and so on. Susan's life has been hurt badly by this behaviour. She needs to either resolve it by reporting the abuse and making sure that the guilty party gets their just desserts, or to move on. It is not her responsibility that the offence occurred and neither is it in any way reasonable that she should suffer the consequences further. Whatever she decides, she must either a report it and move on or not report it and move on. She should also understand that any negative perception she has of herself in the whole affair is wrong and either resolve that fact herself or resolve it with a health professional.

As a career teacher, Susan's perception of the change of duties from research to lecturing classes was very negative, causing her to suffer panic attacks. Yet how many ways can this change in duties be perceived? Presumably research work is relatively isolated and sedentary. A change of duties to teaching classes could well be perceived as a means of moving towards a more active lifestyle. The result being involved more with the students, moving from classroom to classroom, going on field trips and generally being caught up in the general exuberance of youthful students. Susan had put on weight and so a more active lifestyle would almost certainly mean that she would start to lose her excess weight. It is also a perception that mixing with these people will give her the impetus to want to buy better fitting clothes.

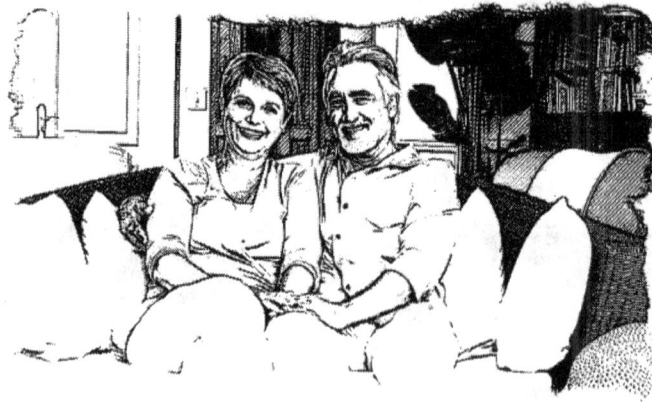

Yet another perception of her change of duties could be that a more active lifestyle would exercise her joints and help her to lose many of the aches and pains she suffered. We could of course go on. Surely it is clear that, without understating the severity of some of the events that had shaped Susan's life and brought her to the depth of suffering that she experienced, so many of these events and her own perceptions of them and not the events themselves had influenced her life. There were a number of alternative perceptions that she could have arrived at, and helping Susan was largely a matter of discussing these different perceptions so that she was able to understand that things did not need to turn out in such a negative fashion as they had.

Susan has not faced up to both her childhood abuse and the difficulties that have troubled her in later life. She made her own decision as to how she would deal with the matter of the abuse and was confident the path she has chosen would be the correct path. We have not asked her what her decision was, that is something that is intensely personal and should she wish is to know it would be up to her to mention it to us. She has made tremendous progress and has now adopted the very sensible practice of writing down anything that occurs in her life that troubles her. She then makes a list of alternative perceptions of what happened so that she can see how to best deal with the matter in a way that offers her the best possible outcome.

In the case of Tony he did, as previously stated, succeed in defeating the cocaine addiction. He took up a regime of healthy exercise as an alternative means of gaining the kind of positive and dynamic outlook which he felt equipped him to do his high pressured managerial career. It emerged that not only had his childhood been bedevilled by the kinds of negative images by people who were not massively successful in their chosen careers, but his whole family were in fact all in high stress high-level occupations. It seemed that the home in he was brought up in was literally a high-pressure cooker just waiting to explode. Sadly Tony was the person chosen to suffer the consequences. Once again, at a very early stage in his life, Tony was equipped with entirely the wrong set of perceptions with which to go forward in life. This warped perception was to influence his thinking right up until the point where his cocaine addiction almost brought him to the very ruin that he had been so frequently threatened with as a child. In some ways the threat of "winding up in the gutter" became a self fulfilling prophecy. Only the understanding of how the complex interactions of his mind and body relative to his physical and mental reactions, as illustrated on the mind compass, gave him the knowledge and understanding to deal with the misinformation he had been equipped with as a child.

Here is a piece that perhaps illustrates the problem of perception more. Because of course changing your perception means changing your attitude, perceiving a factor in your life in a positive way as opposed to a negative way, or perhaps vice versa while you are still struggling with your difficulties. When you can work through your list of perceptions of a particular problem and manage to change your attitude in a way that suits you best, you may consider this short piece.

> "The longer I live, the more I realize the impact of attitude on life. Attitude, to me, is more important than facts. It is more important than the past, than education, than money, than circumstances, than failures, than successes, than what other people think, say or do. It is more important than appearance, giftedness or skill. It will make or break a company, a church, a home. The remarkable thing is we have a choice every day regarding the attitude we will embrace for that day.
>
> We cannot change our past. We cannot change the fact that people will act in a certain way. We cannot change the inevitable. The only thing we can do is play on the one string we have, and that is our attitude. I am convinced that life is 10% what happens to me and 90% how I react to it. And so it is with you. We are in charge of our attitudes. "

> *Rev. Charles Swindoll*

You should now be aware of the whole issue of perception, how we perceive things in different ways and how a single perception of any of the issues and challenges that beset us during our lifetimes is not likely to serve us. Instead, you should be conscious that when you are faced with a problem of any kind, the major or minor, be it a severe panic attack or a simple disagreement with a colleague at work, there are a number of ways that these issues can be perceived. You should be fully aware of these perceptive options and also fully aware when you have jumped to the least helpful or most negative option instead of weighing alternative perceptions of the event before choosing one that is of most benefit to yourself.

Before you proceed to the next chapter write a list. At the head of the list you might say one problem that you feel is affecting your life in a negative way. Under this problem right down your current perception of the difficulty and then make a list of alternative ways that you could perceive the difficulty, concentrating on those ways that will benefit you most.

Fill in the Mood Compass, and keep the chart for future reference.

*Our despondent moods are, for the most part, moods of ingratitude.*

*(unknown)*

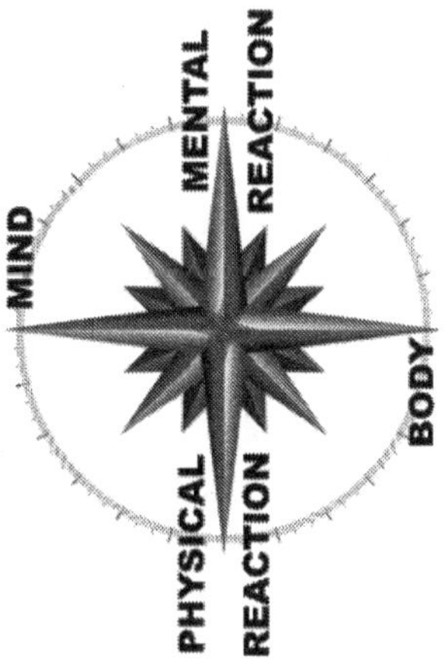
MIND
MENTAL REACTION
BODY
PHYSICAL REACTION

This section continues building upon our understanding of our moods and problems. We will start exploring the West direction of our mood compass in greater detail.

# CHAPTER 3: HEADING WEST

# CHAPTER 3: HEADING WEST

*Certainly there are good and bad times, but our mood changes*
*more often than our fortune*

*Jules Renard*

We are making good progress on the path to understanding and dealing with those unwanted feelings that are draining away the quality of our life. We have explored the various factors that are causing us difficulties and have examined the insidious way in which all of these factors combine to make us feel the way we do. In Chapter 3 we are going to look further to the west of the mind map. This is our mental reactions to stimuli to those events both regular and irregular that we come across on a daily basis and which, if not handled properly, can cause us to increase our suffering.

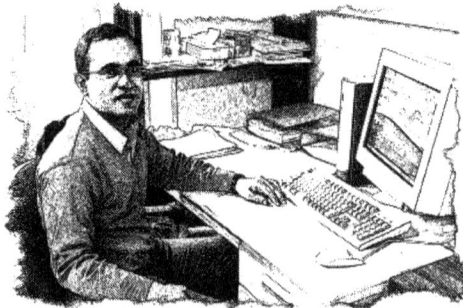

The feeling you experience as a result of any particular stimulus, whether external or internal, we generally call mood. Mood can be a positive or a negative force, depending on the type of mood and of course depending especially on the way we have chosen to perceive the mood in combination with other factors on the mind map. You feel very tired, so tired that the prospect of doing anything active is unattractive to you at this time. Your mood could be very anxious, so anxious that you feel your brain is so numbed that you are unable to make simple decisions when faced with common options. It could even be something as basic and simple as a choice between whether you should go for a healthy and bracing walk, perhaps something you planned yesterday, and watching a programme on the television that may or may not hold some interest for you. When your mood is overly negative it is probably inevitable that you will opt for the least line of resistance, that is the watching television option. For that involves you essentially in not having to make a decision at all. But what is mood? Do we have any labels that we can apply to different moods? The answer is emphatically yes, researchers have identified a great number of different moods.

## MOOD LIST

Acerbic
Aggressive
Ambitious
Amiable/Good-Natured
Angry
Angst-Ridden
Atmospheric
Austere
Autumnal
Bitter
Bittersweet
Bleak
Boisterous
Brash
Brassy
Bravado
Bright
Brittle
Brooding
Calm/Peaceful
Campy
Carefree
Cathartic
Cerebral
Cheerful
Circular
Cold
Complex
Confident
Confrontational
Crunchy
Cynical/Sarcastic
Delicate
Depressed
Detached
Difficult
Distraught
Dramatic
Dreamy
Druggy
Earnest
Earthy
Eccentric
Eerie
Effervescent
Elaborate
Elegant

Energetic
Enigmatic
Epic
Ethereal
Exciting
Exuberant
Fearful
Fierce
Fiery
Fractured
Freakish
Freewheeling
Fun
Gentle
Giddy
Gleeful
Gloomy
Greasy
Gritty
Gutsy
Happy
Harsh
Hedonistic
Hostile
Humorous
Hungry
Hypnotic
Indulgent
Innocent
Insular
Intense
Intimate
Ironic
Irreverent
Joyous
Knotty
Laid-Back/Mellow
Lazy
Light
Literate
Lively
Lush
Malevolent
Manic
Meandering
Melancholy
Miserable

Menacing
Messy
Naive
Nihilistic
Nocturnal
Nostalgic
Ominous
Organic
Outraged
Outrageous
Paranoid
Party/Celebratory
Passionate
Pastoral
Plaintive
Playful
Poignant
Precious
Provocative
Quirky
Rambunctious
Ramshackle
Raucous
Rebellious
Reckless
Refined
Reflective
Relaxed
Reserved
Restrained
Reverent
Rollicking
Romantic
Rousing
Rowdy
Rustic
Sad
Sardonic
Searching
Self-Conscious
Sensual
Sentimental
Sexual
Sexy
Silly
Sleazy
Slick

Smooth
Snide
Soft
Somber
Soothing
Sophisticated
Spacey
Sparkling
Sparse
Spicy
Spiritual
Spooky
Sprawling
Springlike
Stately
Street-Smart
Stylish
Suffocating
Sugary
Summery
Swaggering
Sweet
Tense/Anxious
Theatrical
Thuggish
Tired
Trashy
Trippy
Uncompromising
Unsettling
Urgent
Visceral
Volatile
Warm
Weary
Whimsical
Wintry
Wistful
Witty
Wry
Yearning

This list is by no means definitive. It would be a good exercise for you to take a sheet of paper and make two columns by drawing a line down the centre of the paper, then draw a line across the middle of the page so that you have four quarters. Call the left-hand column positive and the right-hand column negative. In each column put in the various states of mood you can recall feeling in the past seven days. If you are suffering badly with lower mood or some kind of depression, it is likely that the left-hand positive column will be fairly empty, whilst the right-hand negative column will be fuller. That is nothing to be concerned about, because what we want you to do now is in the lower left column write the types of mood that you aspire to feel on a regular basis. Now, when things are looking less favourable than you would prefer, take out this list, we will call it your 'before and after list', and look at the bottom left column. This is the real you. This is what you feel you should be, not the person that dwells on all of the negative things in the top right column. As you progress you will be able to look at the negative moods in the top right column and smile. Whilst when looking at the positive mood in the bottom left column you will begin to feel the dramatic benefits in quality of life that you can experience when these moods are a regular part of your life and your thoughts.

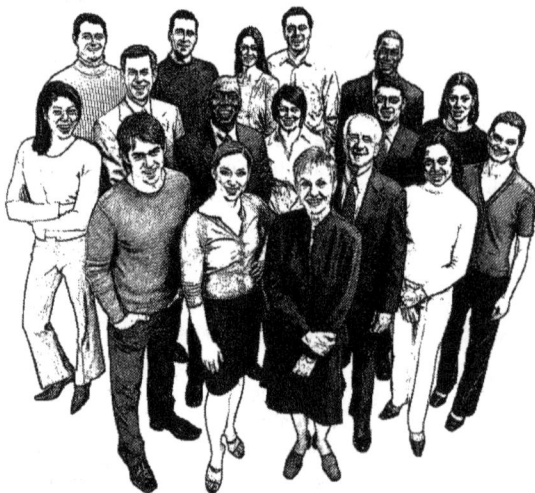

## REMOVING NEGATIVE MOODS

Getting rid of your unwanted negative moods is not something we would want to describe as easy. Just making a list is only the first step on a journey that you are making from darkness into light. Often when you are feeling such negative moods as anxiety, depression, unnecessary tiredness or even headaches and other aches and pains you will find it extremely difficult to identify which particular mood you are experiencing. (Bear in mind that there can be physiological reasons for headaches and aches and pains. If you honestly feel this to be the case, do not hesitate to get them checked out by your doctor.) In short, you just feel rotten. In these situations it is absolutely normal to be unable to identify the source of your problem. At this stage you will almost certainly find it helpful to refer to your list and try to identify exactly just what it is you are experiencing. For example:- What stopped you from going for that walk that you knew would make you feel so good about yourself? Were you too tired? Did you feel anxious or panicky about leaving the house? Perhaps you were nervous about running into a person or situation that you are not fully comfortable with handling? Or did leaving the house just make you feel vaguely unsettled?

We will look at a real-life situation to help with your understanding of the kinds of difficulties that people can face and correctly identifying the cause of their problems. Let's look at Jane, the middle-aged lady in Chapter 1. She had given up her activities because she incorrectly assumed that it was a simple matter of getting old which had caused her to feel less inclined to leave the house and engage in any active leisure pursuits. She was also suffering from insomnia, which she again identified incorrectly as being part of the ageing process. In Jane's case it was quite clear that at no stage had she stopped to consider that there was anything wrong, that there was something specific to her as a person that was causing her such difficulties. These difficulties then resulted in irritability, amongst other things, in dealing with her husband and family.

We now know that the problems Jane was suffering were rather more complex. Ageing was simply an excuse and in this particular case totally incorrect. Going ahead in life with such an incorrect assessment of one's reasons for feeling so tired and disinclined to carry out one's normal activities, or of suffering such a clear and obvious physical symptom as insomnia, is clearly unhelpful. This will only lead to the difficulties being prolonged to the point of destroying any chance of a normal quality of life. But what was Jane's mood when she was feeling so tired and down about everything, or as she described it, "feeling her age"?

One obvious mood she was experiencing at the time was that of being fearful. She was afraid that her husband was in imminent danger of death from a severe

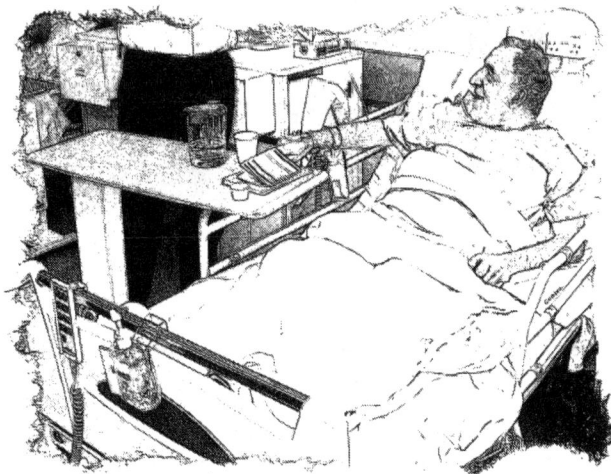

41

heart attack. What else did she feel? Well, gloomy would certainly be one word that comes to mind, possibly distraught. In terms of her normal activities she clearly felt detached. All of these are of course negative moods. In Jane's case were she to make the list of positive and negative moods it would have been fairly clear to her that the reasons for her feeling so tired and elderly was in fact little to do with her actual age in years. On a therapeutic basis we were in fact able to explore with Jane the negative feelings that she was experiencing on a daily basis and examine them one by one, and then in conjunction with the other factors on the mind compass.

Was there any legitimate reason for her to feel so pessimistic about her husband's chances of survival in the face of his mild heart attack? Once the facts known, surely the opposite was true. She had every reason to feel optimistic that a non-life-threatening illness had occurred that served as sufficient warning for him to change his habits so that a major heart attack was substantially less likely, rather than more likely. Yet because of the illness and premature death of her friend from the dance group, she had somehow perceived this as some kind of indication that her husband's life was also in danger.

It was a question of examining her moods, of helping her to seriously question her moods and the reasons for them so that she could understand that her negatives moods were completely unwarranted and unnecessary. She could then look at the more positive moods that she wished to experience ,and in fact had experienced before her friends death, and use them as a road map towards getting back to her old mental state before her husband's illness and friend's death.

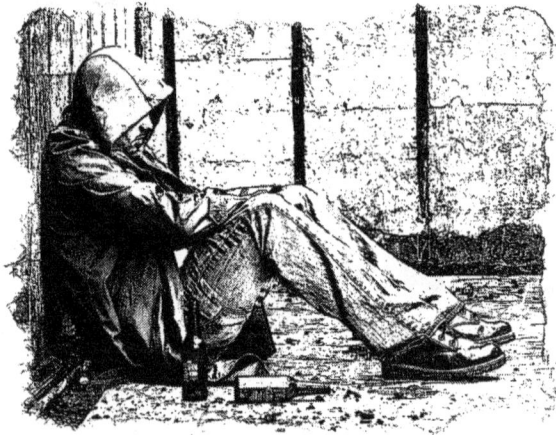

## UNNECESSARILY NEGATIVE MOODS

How does one know when they are experiencing feelings or moods that are unnecessarily negative? Whilst this is not always an easy question to answer, there are some obvious pointers that you can take into account. Apart from the situation in which you find yourself which may give obvious indications of why you are feeling so bad, such as death or illness of a loved one, there are very definite physical indications that you should use as warning signs. If you think about the kinds of physical feelings that occur when you suffer some sort of stressful event these will give you some good pointers in the right direction. For example if you are feeling overly anxious, with or without good reason, it is likely that you will feel your stomach being knotted, as we have previously mentioned. Tightness in the chest is a common feeling when a person is suffering anxiety. Also a numb feeling in the brain is by no means uncommon for anxiety sufferers, including most people experiencing or about to experience a panic attack. Other symptoms can include tingling or numbness in the extremities, soreness in the eyes and of course the major indication of excessive tiredness when there is no good reason for it. If then you feel any of these symptoms, for example you are very tired yet you had a good night's sleep, it is fairly certain that there is something in your mood that is likely to be causing you negative feelings. You would do well to address this as soon as possible. Remember you are beginning to learn the techniques for analysing your mood to give you a good understanding of why you feel the way you do, the way you should be feeling and how to change your mood to a more desirable state.

Tony, the cocaine addict from Chapter 1 frequently found that his feelings were something akin to paranoia. The cocaine had ceased to be effective in any positive sense and was now only taken to feed his addiction. Tony told us of his frequent feelings of sickness and crippling headaches. It is clear that his addiction to a powerful drug was a factor in this problem, but there was certainly more to it than the effect of the drug itself. He was quickly becoming perpetually tearful of his situation at work. This negative mood had no real basis in the actual conditions of his work. The effects of his drug addiction apart, the feelings of sickness and headaches should serve as an indicator that some incorrect assessment of the situation was causing him to become both paranoid and fearful. Were he to write down the negative moods that he was experiencing, together with the positive moods that he remembered experiencing in previous times before he began taking cocaine, he would realise that there was little to be either paranoid or fearful about. Other than the damage he was doing to himself by his drug habit and his incorrect perception of the situation in which he was working.

Put quite simply, deep inside Tony was the same man he had been last year, five years ago and ten years ago. All that had happened was that he had reacted mentally to a series of factors, both real as in the cocaine and imagined as in his ability to do his high-powered job and the derogatory way he felt that his colleagues were viewing him. Once he was able to identify these desperate factors and then look at them all as a whole on the mood compass, he was able to see that (cocaine apart) he was the same man he had always been. Ambitious, hard-working, clever, and talented. The childhood insecurities he had experienced had begun at an early stage to impinge on his mood and instead of dealing with them by recognising how his perception of a given situation was so flawed, he had resorted to cocaine instead with a result that was wholly inevitable.

In a similar way Susan's perception of the given situation is in her day-to-day life, which had been shaped into a large degree by events during her childhood, resulted in her falling victim to panic attacks. Her mood was most certainly fearful with a series of other equally negative moods marking the progress of her days. Once again, her perception of a given situation had been wrongly arrived at as a result of her childhood experiences resulting in a mental reaction, or mood. That only served to lead her further into the depths of misery and despair. During her attacks of panic she told us that she felt unable to breathe. It is important to add at this stage that she did not realise she was suffering from a panic attack. She only thought she was suffering from shortness of breath that caused her to panic, not the reality which was that it was the panic attack itself that was causing her shortness of breath. She blamed the shortness of breath on her putting on weight, which again she blamed was a result of her being unable to breathe freely and without difficulty. Clearly this was a tangled "merry-go-round" and we were able to get her to write down the negative factors she experienced together with the positive factors she wanted to experience. When she had done this she was able to recognise within the list how she felt and reacted before the worst of her panic attacks began to occur. She was also able to recognise how absurd the negative mental reactions were, the moods, when in fact nothing really had changed in her life.

You will see that it is very important to understand your own moods, how you feel at any given time and using the tools you have acquired during the previous chapters to work with your perceptions of mood as a product of understanding or misunderstanding a given situation. The only way we have found for this to be done effectively is for you to write down your experiences. At the same time write down how these experiences affected your mood and do you feel that the effect was reasonable or unreasonable. When a negative mood has affected you badly, how did you feel physically? Did you experience aches and pains in your body, headaches, numbness, shortness of breath?

## YOUR TASKS

Your task for the end of Chapter 3 is to take a sheet of paper and divided into four columns. Using the previous day as your resource, right down your experiences as follows:

- Column 1 - one of your mental reactions or moods that occurred yesterday

- Column 2 - the event that was occurring when you experienced this mood

- Column 3 - how you felt physically at the time in terms of aches, pains, shortness of breath etc

- Column 4 - consider the event you have listed in Column 2 and write what you feel would be a mood, or mental reaction, that would serve you better than the mood you have described in Column 1

Continue with this list using as many different moods as you can recall. Do not just dwell on negative experiences. There is great value in recalling your positive experiences so that you are able to remember readily exactly how you managed to react in such a positive way. In effect you are correcting the negative moods that were an unnecessary result of your perception, for whatever reason, whilst reinforcing those positive experiences that served you best as a person.

Fill in a Mood Compass, and keep it with the previous sheets.

In this chapter we will look in detail at the idea of the mood diary and how it can help you record and monitor your mood. It is important to ensure that you have read and understood the previous 3 chapters before moving on to this section.

# CHAPTER 4: MOOD DIARY

# CHAPTER 4: MOOD DIARY

*One should never criticize his own work except in a fresh and hopeful mood. The self-criticism of a tired mind is suicide.*

*Charles Horton*

During the first three chapters you will have noticed the importance that we place on writing down the things you have experienced. It is important as an exercise because writing these things down enables you to more clearly understand, in strong visual way, exactly what it is that is causing you trouble. If you attempt to sort everything into order in your head, your list is competing with hundreds of thousands of other thoughts that occur to you in the course of a normal day. This is no basis for making a realistic effort to turn your mood around to the point where you become the happy and positive person you want to be.

There are a few basic steps you can take to begin making your list, let's call it a mood diary. The idea of sufferers keeping a mood diary is becoming more and more popular amongst therapists and the various help and self-help groups that exist for sufferers of anxiety and depression related disorders. The consensus is that keeping this kind of written record will be one of the most powerful tools you can use to aid in your recovery from symptoms.

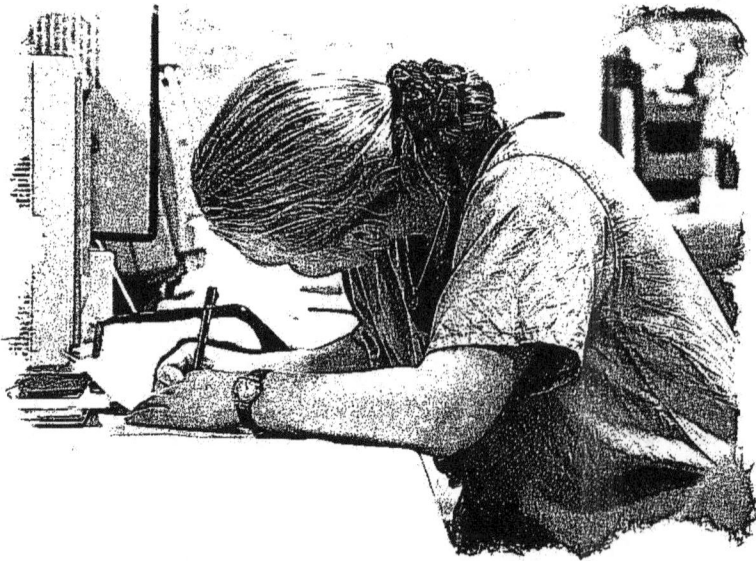

1.  Decide where you want to record your moods - on a calendar, in a spiral notebook, in a journal, on your computer, on an audiocassette/cd you make notes from later. Any system is fine so long as you use one method consistently.

2.  Pick a charting method you think suits you. This can range from simply listing a few descriptive words on a calendar to scoring a mood inventory.

3.  Select the frequency at which you would like to record your moods. If you have long slow cycles, weekly will suffice. If you struggle with rapid cycling bipolar disorder, you will want to do record on a daily basis.

4.  Consider setting a specific time at which to record your feelings. This will help you to remember to do so as well as provide some consistency. Rapid cyclers may want to do so more than once a day.

5.  Record your moods daily or weekly. If you miss a day, try to fill it in as soon as possible.

6.  Note anything significant that may have affected your mood. This could include amount of sleep, a cold, an argument, a rainy day ... and over time, look for patterns that indicate personal triggers.

7.  Keep all of your results together.

8.  Periodically review your charts to note any trends or moods swings.

9.  Share these with your therapist. This will allow him to have a better understanding of how you are really doing and make any necessary adjustments to your treatment.

10. Notify your doctor of any sudden or marked changes in your moods. Early intervention can often nip an episode in the bud!

**TIPS:**

- If you are comfortable with it, you may want to ask a loved one to keep a mood chart for you as well. This will provide another perspective and allow your loved one to feel more involved and helpful.

- Don't punish yourself if you miss charting a day when you are depressed. Instead, note it as a symptom of your mood.

## JANE — DAILY MOOD RECORD     DATE: ......./.............../.............

| Event/Cause | Mood/Mental Reaction | Preferred Mood | Physical Reaction | Preferred Physical Reaction | Body State | Preferred Body State | Mind State | Preferred Mind State |
|---|---|---|---|---|---|---|---|---|
| 3.30am Not sleeping | Fed up | Acceptance | Fidgeting | To feel comfortable | Feet cold | To feel warm and cosy | Anxious | Calm |
| 9.00am Argument with Edward over dress and appearance | Upset | To be realistic and not upset | Tears | No tears | Agitated and pacing up and down | To sit and be comfortable | Angry | Thoughtful |
| 3.30pm Edward's disappearance | Very anxious | Calm | Slightly shaky | To feel normal | Felt hot | Feel comfortable | Very anxious and worried | To feel calm and in control |

# SUSAN — DAILY MOOD RECORD

DATE: .......... / .................. / ..................

| Event/ Cause | Mood/ Mental Reaction | Preferred Mood | Physical Reaction | Preferred Physical Reaction | Body State | Preferred Body State | Mind State | Preferred Mind State |
|---|---|---|---|---|---|---|---|---|
| 8.45 Missed bus | Angry | Accepting — that's life | Pacing up and down | Not to feel so agitated | Warm and flustered | To feel normal | Fed up | To feel happy |
| 12.30 pm Shopping for clothes | Miserable | Enjoying Experience | Red in face | No reaction | Hot and sweaty | Normal Temperature | Embarrassed | Not to care about experience |
| 2.15pm Meeting with senior lecturer about change of job | Felt frightened | Free from Anxiety | Red in face | No reaction | Heart pounding and feel sick | None of this | Out of Control | To be in control |

# TONY  DAILY MOOD RECORD  DATE: ......../.........../.............

| Event/ Cause | Mood/ Mental Reaction | Preferred Mood | Physical Reaction | Preferred Physical Reaction | Body State | Preferred Body State | Mind State | Preferred Mind State |
|---|---|---|---|---|---|---|---|---|
| 7.30am Tanning studio | Acceptance— no choice | No worries | Cold | None | Lethargic | Energetic | Bored | Average |
| 8.30am First visit to gym | Apprehensive and shy | Confident and enjoying experience | Slow and awkward | Active | Hot and uncomfortable | Feel good | Embarrassed | Relaxed |
| 8.30pm Dinner with brother | Miserable and acceptance | Enjoy it for what it is | Agitated | No reaction | Slightly sweaty | Cool and comfortable | Very anxious | Much less anxious |

# DAILY MOOD RECORD

DATE: ........./.............../...............

| Event/ Cause | Mood/ Mental Reaction | Preferred Mood | Physical Reaction | Preferred Physical Reaction | Body State | Preferred Body State | Mind State | Preferred Mind State |
|---|---|---|---|---|---|---|---|---|
| | | | | | | | | |
| | | | | | | | | |
| | | | | | | | | |

## EXAMPLE A

Let's take an example. From the preceding chapters you will have an idea as to the kinds of factors that are an important consideration for your recovery. Remember the mood compass and try to shape your chart so that it will help to form an analysis along similar lines. Bearing in mind the four points of the compass, you can start off with four plus four, or eight columns, as well as a column to the extreme left of the chart. The eight columns will be alternately labelled mood/mental reaction, physical reaction, body state, mind state, with two columns for each factor. To the left of the chart the column is for you to jot down any event that occurred, if any, to bring about that mood state or change of mood.

We now have a chart that looks something like this:

Some of the troubling symptoms we need to be looking for and to address would be such things as:

- excessive, ongoing worry and tension
- an unrealistic view of problems
- restlessness or a feeling of being "edgy"
- irritability
- muscle tension
- headaches
- sweating
- difficulty concentrating
- nausea
- the need to go to the bathroom frequently
- tiredness
- trouble falling or staying asleep
- trembling
- being easily startled

We then need to consider exactly how these symptoms have contributed to our poor mood or lack of wellness. There many aspects of illness and wellness that can create a whole and complete life or the opposite, a miserable and unfulfilled life.

The major areas are:-

- emotional
- intellectual
- physical

- social

- spiritual

- occupational

- environmental

Striking a balance in each of these life areas is what recovery to wellness is all about. This means being aware of each aspect and what role it has in the way we feel.

When there is a breakdown in one area or numerous areas of our wellness, anxiety, panic attacks, mood swings and depression are a common result. The full spectrum of our well-being can run across all aspects simultaneously. When one area is affected other areas are affected as well, whether we realise it or not. Think of them like dominoes. When one falls, others will soon follow. The same is true for the contrary. When we work to raise one aspect of wellness, the others will follow suit. Each of the aspects of wellness are separate on one level, but on another level they are forever interlocked, and it is nearly impossible to practice health in one area without practicing health in the others.

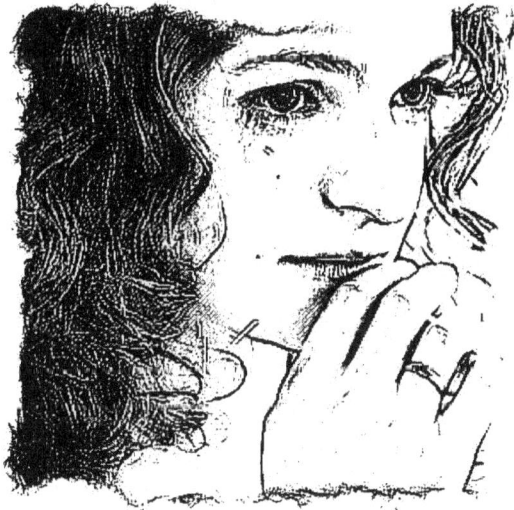

As breakdowns in our wellness occur, anxiety and feelings of depression can become challenges we must face and overcome. Dwelling on past regrets can cause depression, and thinking only about the future can create feelings of uncertainty and anxiety. It's important to try to stay present in the moment. Learning from past mistakes, feeling nostalgia for good times of the past and planning for the future are all helpful. But being present in the here and now is one of the most important things you can do to support your total wellness.

Depression and anxiety can come about quickly and deceptively. Often it seems very hard to get "out of your head" when you're feeling anxious about tomorrow. Depression too, as many of us can attest, causes hopelessness and may be very difficult to overcome. When there is imbalance in the various aspects of wellness, we might begin to feel a sense of lacking. As if we haven't accomplished something or that something is missing in our lives. This can lead to even more breakdowns in our sense of well-being, as feelings of powerlessness or uncertainty keep us from practicing good wellness-related habits in other life areas - such as self-care, chores, friendships and social activities.

It now becomes clear that the chart is an important tool in your recovery. As previously stated, trying to make sense of a number of differing factors, in an already crowded and possibly troubled mind, is not a good way to go forward to recovery. The chart will be your friend, your therapist and your analyst. It will enable you in most cases to make the correct decisions for your recovery, generally by a wider understanding of those factors that have influenced your thinking and are causing you to wrongly perceive events and cause yourself unnecessary suffering.

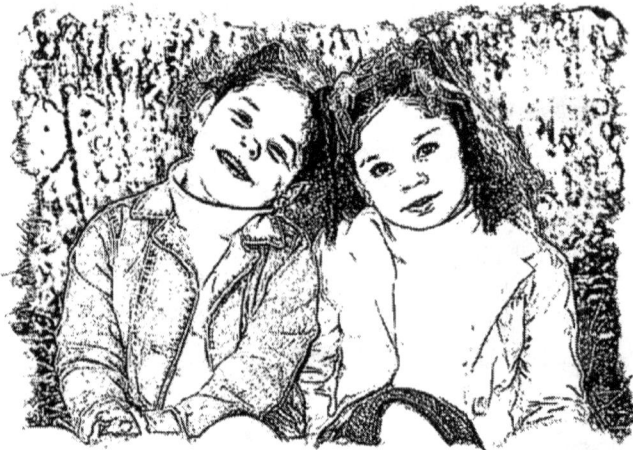

## EXAMPLE B

Here is a typical account of the early life of a child who grew into an adult with the kinds of feelings of poor mood, depression and bipolar disorder that we are working with you to remedy:-

"From a very early age, I can remember being very agitated about some of the smallest things. What's important to a child can of course be nothing of consequence to an adult, but at the time I can remember asking questions that seemed very important to me. Are we late? Is there going to be anybody there? I would be seriously worried about the outcome of the answer to would it rain on school sports day? What would we do? Would it be cancelled? If it didn't rain, would everyone turn up? Did I look ok in my new sports strip? Were we on time? Being late for an occasion opened the door to a whole new set of worries. This sort of worrying may not sound too extreme, but I was only five or six years old.

As far as I can remember, my parents - who 99% of the time were great - never picked up on my excessive anxiety. I always felt fobbed off with a half-baked answer to most of my questions. I honestly feel that if it had been spotted and helped by them, then things may have been easier for me as a child. I'm conscious with my own children today that children need lots of support and lots of love and reassurance from their parents.

One of the more unusual things I used to worry about in my teenage years was the weather. The weather, in particular the wind, used to send shivers down my spine. It caused me to worry and fret about the slightest little thing. As an adult I've done a lot of reading, but have never come across this particular problem - I call it Weather Affective Disorder. It's a close cousin of Seasonal Affective Disorder or SAD, except that while SAD only affects people for a few months of the year, WAD affected me all year round. It could be wind, rain or even the blue sky that bothered me."

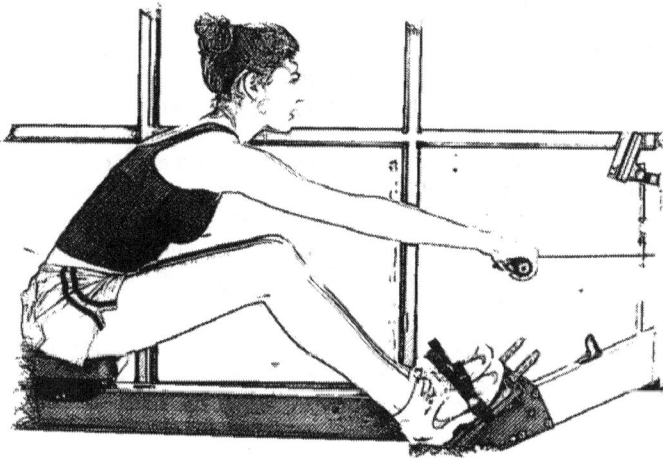

Does any of this sound familiar to you?  Although this person's account does not discuss the reasons for their feelings, clearly they have been excessively negative from a very early age.  It would be almost impossible for this child to grow into an adult without experiencing problems of negative and frequently changing moods.

Why are we recounting this tale?  The answer is that this is all too familiar. Adults looking for therapy invariably can trace their problems back to much earlier times in their lives.  The problem is that may not seem to have been significant at the time but, combined with other factors, is by no means unusual for these kinds of symptoms to develop into negative moods and occasionally clinical depression or bipolar disorder.

There is of course no guarantee that faithfully keeping a mood diary will in itself solve every single one of your problems. We will be looking at a range of other therapies for you to examine and hopefully try out. We will look at these in later chapters. In the meantime you should know that a number of allergy related factors have been linked to severe mood swings. A simple and classic example would be the sugar rush that we have all experienced when eating too much chocolate of sweets. Our mood will be temporarily lifted and then we'll go in the opposite direction, i.e. downwards as the effects of the sugar wear off. Although there are of course physiological reasons for this related to the body's production of insulin we do not need to concern ourselves with the science, simply with cause and effect.

## EXERCISE

Exercise is another important factor that will aid in your recovery. Again we will examine this later in the book. For the time being you should consider how best you can adopt a programme of regular light exercise. Quite apart from the positive effect that exercise has been proved to have on mood, there are the other undoubted benefits of increased cardiovascular fitness and less risk of serious obesity. Family doctors have long recommended exercise as part of a healthy lifestyle and it is one way of maintaining fitness and avoiding obesity.

But does regular exercise really help people manage their troubles? This ia a critical question and one that needs further research. There is a substantial body of scientific research consistently finds that regular exercise is associated with better mood. Meta-analyses show that the effect of exercise is large. That is, exercise can be an effective treatment for mild mood and anxiety problems. In more severe cases it is also helpful in combination with other treatments. In the short-term it can assist with low mood, insomnia and anxiety. In the longer term there are health benefits such as a reduced risk of cardiovascular disease, heart disease, type II diabetes and obesity. Each of these health problems is associated with mood disorders in later life.

There is some debate about the mechanism by which exercise produces psychological benefits. This argument centres on the overall types of exercise and the effects they have on the body. Some researchers have argued that there may be a difference between:-

**AEROBIC EXERCISE - REGULATED BY BREATHING**

- cycling

- running

- walking

- swimming

**ANAEROBIC EXERCISE - WHERE BREATHING IS LESS IMPORTANT**

- weight training

- Pilates

- rock-climbing

Some evidence indicates that aerobic exercise exerts more anti-anxiety effects while anaerobic exercise produces more antidepressant effects. However, more research is needed to clarify these findings.

What is clear is that exercising regularly restores a sense of control that is incompatible with feelings of hopelessness and lethargy that occur in depression. It seems to dissipate stress and anger and assists with anxiety (possibly by disrupting rumination on stressful events).

## TASKS

At the end of Chapter 4 there are two tasks that we would ask you to carry out:-

1. Prepare your own blank mood charts, ideally using a computer for the design of the blank chart so that you can print off charts as and when you need them. The design is entirely up to you and needs to be in the form that is as familiar to you as possible, and therefore easy to use. Alternatively you can use the chart designed earlier in this chapter and make your own version of it. Then prepare three charts, for today, yesterday and tomorrow. Do your best to fill in yesterday's chart with as much as you can remember, fill in today's chart up until now, then keep tomorrows chart to hand and fill it in tomorrow as the day goes through. It would be ideal if you could keep your chart to hand so that as events occur and you feel yourself reacting to them you can jot down the details straightaway without having to worry about forgetting them. Ensure that your charts are all dated and keep them in a folder or ring binder with the latest chart on the top. You will then have an ongoing reference and reminder of the progress you are making and can refer to how you have responded to the events in the past when you feel that you need some kind of guidance or direction.

2. Decide on a simple programme of daily exercise, the simpler the better. If you are unwilling or unable to do anything too ambitious, make a resolution to always use stairs instead of lifts and escalators. Make a decision to walk a short distance of perhaps a few hundred yards when you may normally be tempted to take the car. At a later stage, you may find yourself able to remember the joy and happiness of some kind of hobby or sport that you used to do and have since forgotten about. In the case of Jane, the middle-aged lady we introduced you to in Chapter 1, she was delighted she was able to resume them when she had recovered and found an almost immeasurable amount of happiness and joy. However, the rule here is keep it short, keep it simple, do not become too ambitious. A short walk or run up the stairs could be plenty to start with. Remember, this is something that you have achieved, perhaps

a tiny something, but more than you were doing before. Enjoy that feeling of achievement, remember it, and remember how you got it. Then, when you are ready, go out and look for more of it!

3. As before, fill in another Mood Compass and keep it together with the previous ones. Look at the sheets you have done. Can you see any changes, hopefully improvements?

*The thing with pretending you're in a good mood is that sometimes you can.*

*Charles de Lint*

This part of the book is focused very clearly on your thoughts and feelings. You will find that these core thoughts are based on a variety of things including your automatic thoughts as well as well as the world in which you live.

# CHAPTER 5: THOUGHTS

# CHAPTER 5: THOUGHTS

*At first, I only laughed at myself. Then I noticed that life itself is
amusing. I've been in a generally good mood ever since.*

Marilyn vos Savant

Our thoughts create our feelings, and our feelings cause us to behave the way we do. Most of the thoughts that we have in any given situation are called automatic thoughts. They're referred to as "automatic" because we don't create them. They are based on beliefs we have about ourselves and the world in which we live. When we understand how our automatic thoughts create our feelings and, in turn our behavior, we can seek to change our automatic thoughts by changing our deeply-held core beliefs.

When we are in any situation thoughts about what is going on around, and inside of us, are flying through our heads. If someone cuts us up in traffic we may have an automatic thought - that is so rude and dangerous! This thought will then spark a feeling of anger. If we feel angry, we may scream and yell in our car, catch up with the person and point angry gestures. Or even take that anger home and shout at our loved ones. That single automatic thought starts a chain reaction that upsets us and possibly the people around us. We think that our automatic thought is right, but there are actually many different thoughts that we might have in the same situation.

Automatic thoughts are just what the name implies. They are the thoughts that occur constantly as our minds seek to narrate what is going on around us. The limbic system is the area of the brain that controls immediate response to situations, and this is where our automatic thoughts are born. It assesses what is going on quickly and makes a snap judgment based on the information at hand.

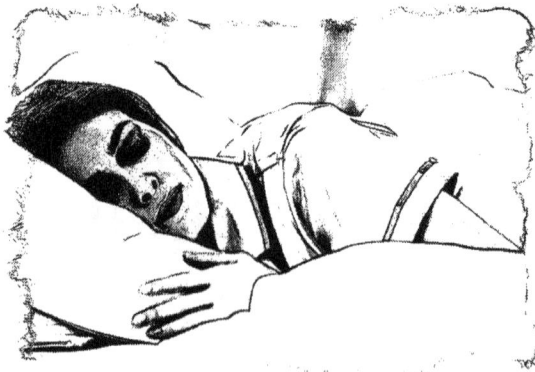

This is very helpful in situations where a quick response is desired, such as an emergency or crisis. In other situations though, it would be better for us to slow down and wait for more information and not react to situations based on our limbic system's messages alone. If left unchecked automatic thoughts may lead to emotional wellness concerns as anxiety, depression, stress and sleep difficulties.

Everything we think is an automatic thought. A problem arises when our automatic thoughts manifest as cognitive distortions. Cognitive distortions are automatic thoughts that are based on deeply ingrained core beliefs. They are irrational reactions we habitually have to situations. We often don't even know that we see the world in terms of these cognitive distortions. Just as the name implies, they are based on faulty reasoning. There are several types of common cognitive distortions.

As we go through life we learn from our experiences. It is a natural process of trial and error. Problems arise when we lump all similar experiences together and decide that all experiences of a certain nature will always turn out the same way. See the uses of the words "all" and "always" in that last sentence? That's a hint at overgeneralisation. If Jane was dumped by her first boyfriend and decided from then on that she is destined to always get dumped, she'd be making an overgeneralisation. This thinking doesn't take into account the different factors that affect every situation. Instead of assessing why she was dumped by her first boyfriend and learning from the actual experience as it happened, she simply decided to learn a general lesson about the nature of relationships. This can obviously lead to trouble. As she goes through relationships later in life operating under this assumption, she'll be much more likely to act in ways that will fulfill her fears. She won't be able to open up and communicate in her relationships because she won't be comfortable. This will lead to more experiences of being dumped, and if she continues to overgeneralise, this will just reinforce the assumption. It will also prevent her from learning about the subtle intricacies of her experiences.

## LABELLING

Labelling is similar to overgeneralisation. It can take the form of making sweeping overgeneralisations about a group of people based on the actions of only a few of them. It can also manifest as self-labelling. Self-labelling can have extremely negative effects. If a person has a bad grade on a maths test and automatically says, "I'm a bad maths student", they won't take the steps necessary to improve their maths skills. "Bad maths student" is a label that they've applied to themselves, and it most likely is not true. With further study, this person would be able to figure out what they did wrong and how to do it right. Instead, by labelling themselves as a "bad maths student", they do not have to take responsibility for doing the work to learn about maths. These labels are self-defeating, and they often lead us to create the very situation that is causing us problems.

Often we assume that we know what people are thinking about us, even if their actions are neutral or indicate the contrary. This is referred to as mind reading. Most people accept that we cannot really read minds. If we're having a conversation with somebody and they correct us about something, we are

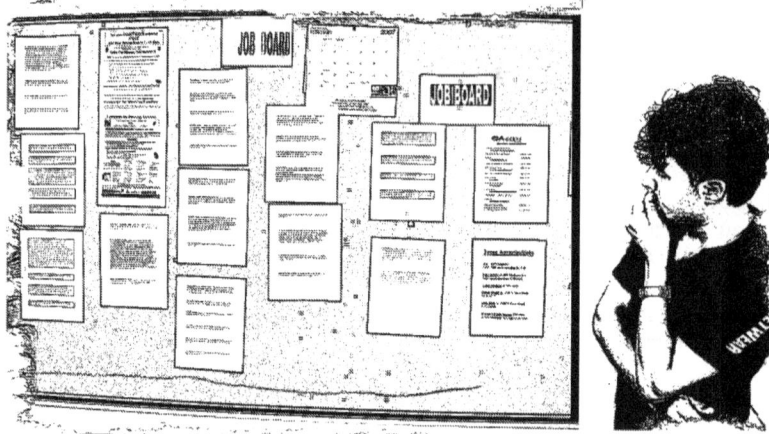

likely to automatically think, "Oh, no, they think I'm an idiot!" This is probably not true. We are much more critical of ourselves than others are of us. In fact, they probably didn't even think anything at all about our mistake. Yet we will let what we assume they think about us affect our behavior for the rest of our conversation with that person and this might make for some negative outcomes as we assume they thought the worst of us.

When we assume we know what will happen in the future we're fortune telling.

## EXAMPLE

Dave is looking for a job. Every time he sits down to send out resumes he thinks, "There's no way I'm even going to get considered for these jobs." He sends out the resumes anyway, but never follows up with a phone call or tries to set up any interviews. Because he's automatically assumed that he won't get the jobs he doesn't try very hard to stand out from the other applicants. He's convinced they're better than him. His fortune telling in this situation prevents him from putting in any effort. Not surprisingly, he doesn't get the jobs, but it's because his negative fortune telling is controlling his behavior.

Often we try to predict the future in situations without any evidence to support our claim, and sometimes we even try to predict an outcome when there's evidence to the contrary. Negative fortune telling without proper objective evidence sets us up for failure because we'll be much less likely to give the situation the chance it deserves.

As we've seen, sometimes our automatic thoughts are based on irrational assumptions. If we stop and think about them rationally, breaking them down based on solid evidence, then we see them as irrational and replace them with new, more rational viewpoints. If we analyse them with emotional reasoning though, we feed into them and come to faulty conclusions. Basically, emotional reasoning is basing our thoughts and beliefs on our feelings. If you're getting ready to give a speech in a meeting and you're nervous, you might think, "I must not be very well prepared. Otherwise I would not be so nervous. I am going to make a fool out of myself!" Even though you spent several hours the day before preparing materials and information for this presentation, you are discounting this fact because you are nervous about speaking in front of your boss and co-workers. Nervousness is a normal emotional reaction to the situation, but it doesn't mean that you don't know the material. This reasoning doesn't work because the only evidence used is the way you feel in a certain situation, and it doesn't take into account all the other factors operating at the time.

"Shoulding yourself" is criticising yourself by concentrating on all the things you should be doing instead of whatever you are doing at the time. If you are watching a movie and all you can think is, "I should be studying/cleaning the kitchen/walking the dog." You diminish any possible enjoyment you could be getting out of watching the movie. You also make it much less likely that you'll actually do all those things you "should" be doing. By simply saying, "I should be studying" you make it into a chore completely devoid of any benefit, and you won't want to do it. If instead you think, "If I study now I will have more time tomorrow to hang out with my friends, and I'd rather hang out with them tomorrow than watch this movie right now." Then you are weighing your options and making a decision to study that will yield a positive result. Sure, everyone has obligations in situations they have to take care of, and these obligations are not always exactly what we would like to be doing at the time. By weighing the costs and benefits, rather than simply imposing "shoulds" on every situation, we can make the most of our time and get more enjoyment out of life. Some shoulds are even more harmful. "I should be studying" will most likely just lead to procrastination. "I should be reading a classic novel by Dickens, rather than this sci-fi fantasy fiction because I need to get smarter." is worse because it is based on the idea that we should spend even our free time doing what other people expect of us. Or, in many cases what we think they expect of us, rather than what we enjoy or think is right. A great example is people who go to college because they think that they "should." If, after weighing all the options, someone decides that college is not the best option for them, they don't have to go even if they think that others will judge them for that choice. "Shoulding" ourselves can lead to making major life decisions that are not necessarily the actual best choices.

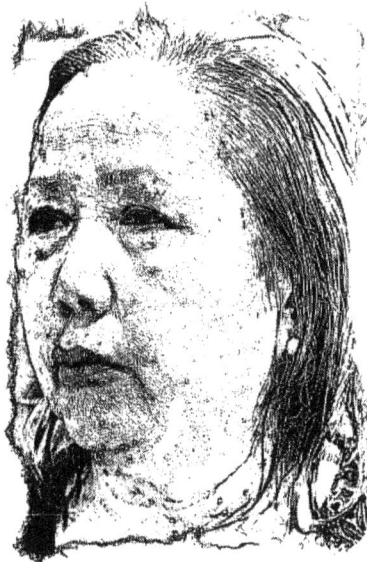

## PERSONALISATION

Personalisation is when we take the blame for outcomes that are beyond our control. Blame is when we point the finger at somebody else for an outcome something that we caused. Personalisation and blame are both based on the assumption that people should be perfect and never make mistakes. When mistakes are made, someone must be at fault and made to pay. The problem here is that everybody makes mistakes. Mistakes are simply an opportunity for us to learn to be better and grow. Punishment is not necessary for everyday errors. The idea is to see where we went wrong and try to do better in the future. It also means learning to distinguish between things we did wrong, factors we couldn't control (such as other people's reactions, opinions, and ideas), and things that were caused by other's actions. Let's say that Jane, who was dumped a few examples ago, she was dumped because her boyfriend was moving away and didn't want to try maintaining a long distance relationship. If she tells herself, "I don't care what he says. I got dumped because I'm ugly and stupid". She's then blaming herself for the outcome of a situation, when it actually had nothing to do with who she is. It was not her fault that he had to move, and it was not her fault that he does not believe in long distance relationships. Now she feels guilty for being herself (which by the way, is not "ugly" or "stupid"—these are cognitive distortions).

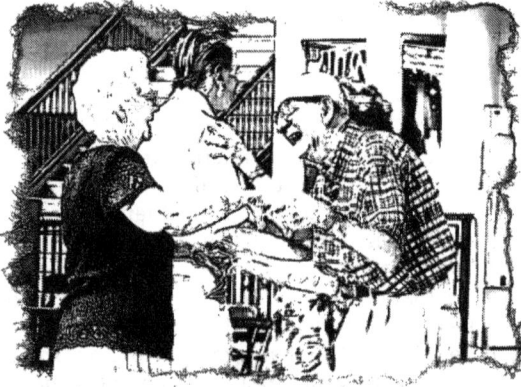

All-or-nothing thinking is the same as saying, "Everything is black or white". Perfectionists often engage in all-or-nothing thinking. People are either all good or all bad. An example would be if Bob overslept one morning and thought, "I don't have time to run my usual full five miles today, so I'm not going to run at all. I'm so lazy". Even though Bob does have time to run three miles, he's given up because he cannot see the benefit in modifying his standard. He also has decided that this automatically makes him a bad person. Many times women will engage in all-or-nothing thinking about their bodies. They think, "Either I am thin, toned, and a perfect size 6, or I'm a fat disgusting slob in a size 10". This is a distortion. It does not take into account that people are different. There are variations in height, frame and muscular structure that can influence our size. This one example of all-or-nothing thinking can lead to more harmful thinking such as, "I'm already fat, so I might as well just eat that whole pint of ice cream and tin of biscuits". Or another extreme, "I'm so fat, I should only eat an apple at breakfast, lunch, and dinner". All-or-nothing thinking looks at things as absolutes rather than a combination of factors. It also assumes that people, places and things can be perfect, and if they're not completely without flaws they must be horrible.

All of these cognitive distortions can have harmful effects on our feelings and behaviour. By learning to recognise them, we can learn to talk ourselves out of such thinking and see things in a more positive light. They will not go away just because we realise they are there, but we can learn how to spot them when they do arise and change our outlook by applying more rational thinking.

Let's look at Jane, the middle-aged lady who was afraid of her husband dying prematurely from a heart attack. The behaviour that prompted her husband Edward to persuade her to speak to a therapist was ultimately her constant irritability, principally with him. He would say to her "Darling, are you going to get back to your dancing classes this week?". The automatic thoughts that would rushed through her brain were concern that if she was several miles away conducting a dance class in senior citizens centre her husband might be lying on the floor dying from a heart attack, gasping out his last breath while she was too far away to help. Surely he realised the problem, the danger that he was in? Did he want to die prematurely like her friend? Why was he suggesting that she leaves the house for several hours at a time and go to a dancing class that was essentially frivolous compared to the real concern of being at home in case anything happened. Was he trying to get rid of her?

These were the automatic thoughts in her mind and she would reply with an irritable retort. "Don't be so stupid Edward, I've got much more important things on my plate. Just leave me alone to get on with things." The reality of course was quite different. Her husband Edward deserved full marks for his efforts to get his wife back into the old routine that had given her such a happy and fulfilling life. He was concerned at her increasingly low state of mood and poor grooming that was, he knew, nothing whatever like the woman that his wife really was.

It would be normal behaviour for the majority of people to be pleased when their partner took some interest in them. Clearly there was no good reason for Jane not carrying on with her activities as she used to. In fact it would be fair to say that she could consider herself much freer to go and pursue those activities, given that the hidden danger that her husband was in had been dealt with. He was in a much healthier state than he had been, because of changes they have made in his lifestyle, and consequently at considerably less risk than before. This however is objective thinking. Automatic thoughts are anything but objective. They are the kinds of thoughts that pop into the mind unannounced, when the person's mood is low. The automatic thought will inevitably reflect that mood, hence Jane's automatic reply. Automatic thoughts are often situation specific instances of more core fixed beliefs about yourself and the world. While automatic thoughts reflect your reaction to a given event, core beliefs describe your general expectations and identity. For example, if you have recently done poorly on a test your automatic thought will probably reflect your situation, "I'm so embarrassed! I should have done better". While your core belief might reflect a deeper fear, "I'm a stupid person". Core beliefs influence appraisals, and thus are a major source of bias. They are not always obvious or conscious. The way to identify them is to examine multiple instances of your automatic thoughts over time for the repetitive themes that underlie them. You will likely be able to distill some of your core beliefs by examining your self-monitoring thought records, and by asking yourself the question, Why am I reacting this way?

We have prepared a questionnaire view to fill in that will help you to analyse the automatic thoughts that pop into your mind. This will be your self-monitoring thought record. It is entirely up to you as to how many of these records you wish to keep. Some people may prefer to keep a daily record, others would feel a less frequent record, such as weekly, would be more useful. We would suggest at the outset you use a separate sheet or record for each day so that you can get into the habit of writing down and monitoring your own thoughts.

# JANE — DAILY THOUGHT RECORD

DATE: ......../........../..............

| Event/ Cause | Mood/ Mental Reaction | Thought (s) | Reason for this thought | Why is this thought realistic? | Why is this thought unrealistic? | What SHOULD I have thought? | Mind State | Do I feel better now about this situation? |
|---|---|---|---|---|---|---|---|---|
| Shopping | Anxious | Is Edward ok? | He might be ill | Because he has been ill before | He has recovered well with no further health problems | It's nice to be out | Still anxious | A little |
| Going to Hairdresser | Fed up | Why bother with this? | No point— getting older | Because I am getting older | No reason to let myself go | Nice to be fussed over | Not feeling confident | No |
| Dancing visit to local senior citizens club | Very nervous | What if Edward is taken ill? Can't get back in time? | So worried he might have another heart attack and die | Because I am worried about him | He's better now | I've missed dancing and going out | Unsure of Myself | A little |

70

THOUGHTS

SUSAN  DAILY THOUGHT RECORD  DATE: ......../......../........

| Event/ Cause | Mood/ Mental Reaction | Thought (s) | Reason for this thought | Why is this thought realistic? | Why is this thought unrealistic? | What SHOULD I have thought? | Mind State | Do I feel better now about this situation? |
|---|---|---|---|---|---|---|---|---|
| Zip broke on dress | Distraught | I am a complete failure | I'm fat | I have put on so much weight | It's not | I don't know | Bad | No! |
| Sunday evening— preparing for work Monday am | No point in this | I can't do this | I'm no good at this | The students will think I am useless | I don't think it is | I can do this | Very anxious | Still no! |
| Joined a slimming club | Shame and embarrassment | Why has it all gone wrong? | Nothing is working for me | I'm not coping | I've made the first move—to lose weight | I can do this, I won't be on my own | Worried | Just a little |

TONY    DAILY THOUGHT RECORD    DATE: ......../.................../........

| Event/ Cause | Mood/ Mental Reaction | Thought (s) | Reason for this thought | Why is this thought realistic? | Why is this thought unrealistic? | What SHOULD I have thought? | Mind State | Do I feel better now about this situation? |
|---|---|---|---|---|---|---|---|---|
| Dinner with relatives | Felt wound up | Will they talking about work etc all evening | They always do—and criticise | It's true | Maybe I let them | I'll try to control the conversation more | Acceptance | No |
| First visit to the gym | Pleased but Apprehensive | This is good | Positive for once | It is | It's not | The same | Almost happy | Yes |
| Taking cocaine | No change | This is not good | It is making things worse | It is making things worse | It's not | Why do I do this? | Not in Control | Just a bit |

THOUGHTS

# DAILY THOUGHT RECORD DATE: ......../............../............

| Event/ Cause | Mood/ Mental Reaction | Thought (s) | Reason for this thought | Why is this thought realistic? | Why is this thought unrealistic? | What SHOULD I have thought? | Mind State | Do I feel better now about this situation? |
|---|---|---|---|---|---|---|---|---|
| | | | | | | | | |
| | | | | | | | | |
| | | | | | | | | |

When Susan was directed to start teaching class again the automatic thoughts that popped into her head were – "I can't do this, they'll all be laughing at me", "If I have to stand in front of that class I will freeze up and look like a total idiot", "and "I'm just not good enough to teach a class full of students, I'm not a very good person". - The next thoughts that occasionally came to mind during this period were to blame the students for not being sympathetic, for being critical and cruel. This of course before she had even met them or stood in front of the class! What was necessary was for Susan to acquire a more cognitive understanding of what she was thinking and analyse her thoughts so that she could understand how irrational they were. It follows from here that she can work out and adjust her thoughts and thought processes so that she is able to respond to stimuli and events as they occur in a way that is more reasonable and fitted to the nature of the occurrence. In this particular example, if she was to read this account of her automatic thought process she would of course realise how unsuitable it was. Thus she would be able to frame responses that were more realistic and help herself to mend her mental reactions or moods to return her quality of life to a much happier state.

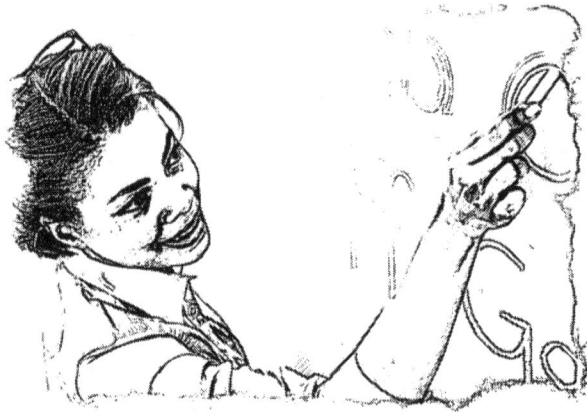

Tony was a clever man, well educated and holding down a prestigious job. When the pressure of his job began piling up he automatic thought was - "There's no way I can do this, I need a boost to get me through". This was the beginning of the path to his destructive cocaine habit. He also thought "These younger people think I'm past it, that I can't handle the pressure of work, they're just waiting for me to fall so that they can step into my shoes." The reality was of course quite different. Tony did manage to do the job efficiently and well. The only real and substantive difficulty arrived when his cocaine habit got out of hand. The truth is that he had been given the job because of his proven worth and ability in that type of work. As for the younger people he worked with, after discussing the problem, he did agree that there was no actual evidence that they were anything other than normally ambitious young people. They may well have wanted to step into his job but only in the normal course of promotion. There was actually no evidence whatsoever that they had displayed any kind of negative behaviour towards him. Their only behaviour had been that of a normal friendly working relationship.

# THOUGHTS

Writing down your automatic thoughts and core beliefs makes it easier for you to view them from an outsider's perspective rather than your own. When you actually look at what you are thinking and believing, you may find that your thoughts and beliefs are inaccurate, incorrect or irrational. With some work you can correct them so that they better reflect "reality", the shared social consensus. Thoughts are mental behaviors typically taking the form of unspoken conversations, running commentaries, visual images or sounds. They are continuous and constant, always occurring in one form or another throughout our lives. Sometimes we are aware of thoughts, and sometimes we are unaware. We can control them when we choose, but we cannot turn them off. When we are not controlling thoughts ourselves, they are controlling us. Thoughts exert a profound influence on how we feel and what we do. Because thoughts are a type of behaviour, albeit a hidden or covert sort of behaviour, they can be manipulated by using methods derived from learning theory.

According to the cognitive behavioural model (a highly regarded approach to psychotherapy derived from learning theory), thoughts are like a lens through which you examine and make sense of the world. Events that happen have no inherent meaning. Instead you assign meaning to the events you experience through a process known as appraisal, which is a fancy word for judgment. In essence, when something happens, you think about that thing and then figure out what that thing means for you and your life; whether it is good or bad. Your judgments end up having rewarding or punishing properties, depending on whether you think things are good or bad, respectively. The thing that is punished or rewarded most primarily is your mood. Rewarding thoughts (positive appraisals) enhance your mood and punishing thoughts (negative appraisals) tend to depress or make you anxious.

There is a school of thought that suggests repeating affirmations to oneself can be a very useful and valuable practice in overcoming the negative aspects of automatic thoughts. The simplest approach to self-suggestion involves simply repeating a new idea about yourself to yourself on a regular basis. Most typically this exercise takes the form of affirmations designed to increase self-esteem, such as "you are a good and decent person". Team chants are designed to motivate or increase team spirit. Any statement may be repeated, however. The idea is based on learning theory again, although loosely in this simple form. By repeating the statement again and again, you are conditioning yourself to learn the statement. Whether or not you will start to believe that the statement is true is another thing entirely.

Self-monitoring exercises help you to become aware of your triggers and the other rewards and punishers in your environment that control your habit. Once aware of these influences you have the opportunity to alter them, or your susceptibility to them. If you succeed in avoiding your habit for long enough it will naturally weaken in strength, due to a process called extinction, and you will ultimately become free of it. This is much easier said than done, of course.

In order to start yourself on this road to self-monitoring it is essential for you to begin using a thought monitoring chart. We have put in examples of thought monitoring charts from our three subjects, Jane, Susan and Tony. These are actual charts that were produced during the early period of their therapy and all proved to be very valuable in their recovery.

## TASK

Your task at the end of Chapter 5 therefore is to produce your own blank thought monitoring chart using the examples in this chapter as a basis for your design. Ideally you would do this on a computer so that charts could be printed out as and when you need them. However if you prefer you could draw the chart by hand and just photocopy them as necessary. Start doing this exercise on a daily basis, and keep to this daily schedule, until such time as you begin to feel more comfortable with the automatic thoughts that pop into your head in any given situation, especially those situations that have caused you difficulty in the past.

As before, fill in a further Mood Compass and keep it with the previous ones. Whenever possible, take the time to compare these to give you an indicator of your progress.

*Faith is the art of holding on to things your reason has once accepted in spite of your changing moods*

*C.S. Lewis*

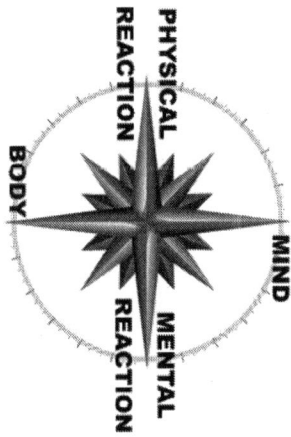

PHYSICAL REACTION

BODY

MIND

MENTAL REACTION

This part of the book introduces the important ideas of using different types of exercise and training regimes to alter and improve your mood and lifestyle. This chapter can be truly life changing for all!

# CHAPTER 6: EXERCISE

# CHAPTER 6: EXERCISE

*The pursuit of happiness, which American citizens are obliged to undertake, tends to involve them in trying to perpetuate the moods, tastes and aptitudes of youth.*

*Malcolm Muggeridge*

Numerous studies have found aerobic exercise works as effectively as antidepressants. Generally, the last thing you want to do when you're depressed is exercise, but even a five minute walk can help. Exercise restores regular sleep and eating, raises energy levels, generates endorphins, boosts serotonin levels and may stimulate new brain cell growth.

Studies have shown that exercise may provide an immediate mood boost for people suffering from depression. Although previous studies have suggested that exercise programmes can take weeks to improve depressive symptoms, a new study suggests that even a single workout can provide immediate benefits in lifting the mood of the seriously depressed.

"Many people with depression attempt to self-medicate with alcohol, caffeine or tobacco to manage their daily routine. Low to moderate intensity exercise appears to be an alternate way to manage depression, one that doesn't come with such negative health consequences." researcher John Bartholomew PhD says in a news release. Bartholomew is an associate professor in the Department of Kinesiology and Health Education at The University of Texas Austin.

Researchers say most research on depression and exercise has focused on exercise as a treatment for the underlying disorder of depression. Instead this study looked at whether exercise might also provide more immediate short-term benefits by lifting people's mood. In the study researchers compared the effects of thirty minutes of walking on a treadmill, with thirty minutes of quiet rest, in forty adults recently diagnosed with depression. None of the participants was taking antidepressants or exercising regularly.

The results showed that both groups reported reductions in feelings of tension, anger, depression and fatigue. But only the exercise group reported feeling good, as measured by improved scores on "vigour" and "well-being" indicators.

The following components are essential to a safe, effective cardiovascular exercise programme. While this sets a foundation for training it is not an exclusive list. New exercisers are encouraged to have a check-up and get a doctor's approval before beginning an exercise programme.

Firstly, determine your maximum heart rate. While there

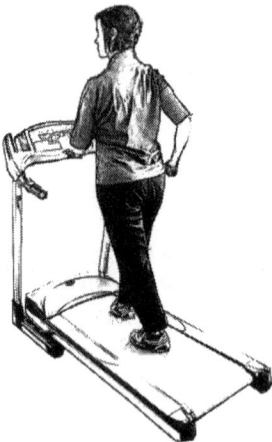

are complicated treadmill tests to objectively measure maximum heart rate, most people will use a simple calculation to estimate maximum heart rate. The easiest formula is simply to subtract your age from 220. A new method, published in the Journal of the American College of Cardiology, estimates maximum heart rate with the following formula:-

208 minus 0.7 times age

Now that you know your maximum heart rate you will determine your overall training goal, and set your exercise intensity accordingly.

## INTENSITY

Determining how hard to exercise is the basis for solid training. Intensity simply refers to your heart rate during training. The appropriate exercise intensity depends upon your maximum heart rate, your current level of fitness and your goals.

## TRAINING ZONES

- If you are just starting an exercise programme it is essential that you check with your doctor before beginning. After you get the go-ahead, it is recommended that you exercise between 50 - 60 percent of your maximum heart rate.

- If you already exercise regularly and would like to continue increasing overall fitness, or improve your times, you should exercise at 60 - 70 percent of maximum heart rate.

- If your goal is to improve aerobic capacity or athletic performance, you will likely be exercising in the training zone which is 75 - 85 percent of maximum heart rate.

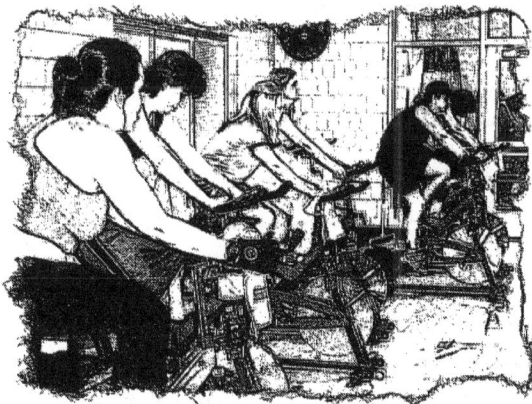

While these zones are general recommendations, it is important to understand that varying your training intensity is important no matter what your fitness level. There may be times when a highly trained athlete will train in the 50 - 60 percent zone (for recovery or long, slow, distance training, for example). Studies show that people who exercise at too high an intensity have more injuries and are more likely to give up.

## TYPE OF EXERCISE

For general conditioning choose activities that use large muscle groups and which are continuous in nature. Some good examples are walking, swimming, running, aerobic dance, stair climbing machines, ski machines, treadmills, cycling or exercise bikes.

For those who are seeking to improve athletic performance, you will also want to use sport-specific training. The principle of specificity states that to become better at a particular exercise or skill, you must perform that exercise or skill. Therefore, a runner should train by running and a swimmer should train by swimming. There are however, some good reasons to cross train, and it is recommended for all athletes.

You should bear in mind that initially you are not looking to win a gold medal in the next Olympic Games. Your goal is to recover from problems associated with low mood and its related illnesses, including depression, bipolar disorder and anxiety. As we stated previously, you need to begin at the lowest possible level. Just walking up the stairs to your office is instead of using the lift could be very difficult for you if you have spent many years in a sedentary lifestyle and you are very unfit. It may be that you are suffering from the effects of obesity, which in itself presents a possible risk when you are embarking on a programme of exercise. As stated, if you plan to embark on a programme of exercise make sure that you get yourself checked out first. Getting yourself on the road to recovery from a severe mood disorder only to collapse with a heart attack would clearly be self-defeating, and could even result in premature death.

The good news is that the vast majority of people are able to find their lives massively enhanced when they begin a modest programme of exercise. People that have suffered from mood disorders find that their darkest moods begin lifting and becoming lighter. They find that their outlook on life and general enthusiasm for life steadily improves. Those people that are obese will inevitably find that there weight will begin to normalise. In fact, providing that you are otherwise fit and healthy there is absolutely no reason why you should not embark straightaway on a limited exercise programme.

Again, assuming that everything else is equal, and that you do not suffer from adverse indications, there is absolutely no downside to an exercise programme. You will feel better, look better and inevitably begin to lose some of the effects of ageing. On a simple level, somebody that lives a sedentary lifestyle is likely to be hunched and stooped in their posture with the inevitable "hangdog" expression that you will see in these people. The next time you are in a commercial area, which will certainly have a substantial population of middle-aged desk bound office workers, look for the fatter middle-aged and younger people that you come across. Look at the hunched rounded shoulders, and the expression on their faces which is generally anything that optimism and enthusiasm for the life they are leading and planned to lead in the future. In a before and after scenario you have now looked at the before. What we are intending to help you achieve is the after scenario. Upright posture, normal weight and an expression that says that this person is confident about the life they are leading and are planning for the future. It is this kind of result that we are looking to achieve by beginning to supplement your development in understanding and perceiving why you feel the way you do in certain situations. Remember the mood compass. The southerly point of the compass is the description of the way your body feels, which is of course is strongly influenced by your reactions both mental and physical and the resultant moods that you experience from these reactions. But at the same time your body is the whole foundation of your life. Put in its simplest terms, the fitter and healthier you are, the happier you will feel and the more options you will have available to you as you go through life.

Do you need more convincing of the benefits of exercise? The average adult has two to three upper respiratory infections each year. We are exposed to bacteria all day long, but some people seem more susceptible to catching the bug. The following factors have all been associated with impaired immune function and increased risk of catching colds.

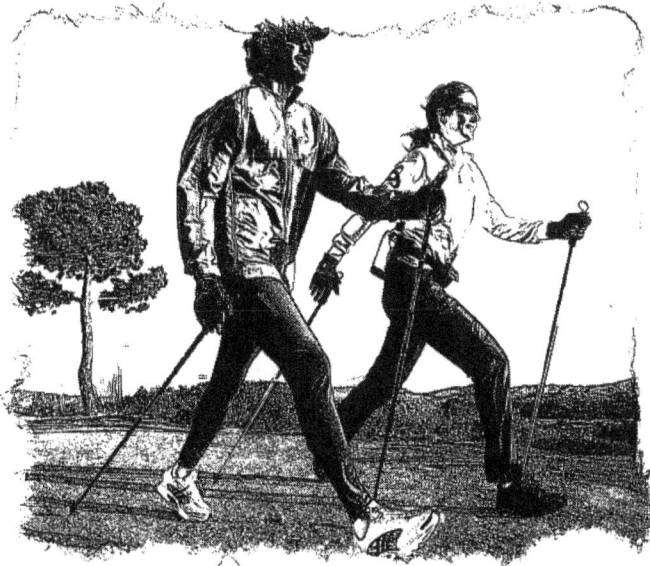

TONY

| ACTIVITY | Mon. | Tues. | Wed. | Thurs. | Fri. | Sat. | Sun. |
|---|---|---|---|---|---|---|---|
| Brisk Walking | | | | | | | |
| Gardening | | | | | | | |
| Mowing lawn | | | | | | | |
| Stretching Exercises | ✓ | | | | | | |
| Weight Lifting | | ✓ | | ✓ | | ✓ | |
| Jogging/ Running | ✓ | | | | | | |
| Aerobics | | | | | | | |
| Bicycling | | | | | | | |
| Stair Climbing | | | | | | | |
| Swimming | | | | | | | |
| Tennis | | | | | | | |
| Bowling | | | | | | | |
| Golf | | | | | | | |
| Other Sports | | | | | | | |
| Dancing | | | | | | | |
| Other Activities | | | | | | | |

SUSAN

| ACTIVITY | Mon. | Tues. | Wed. | Thurs. | Fri. | Sat. | Sun. |
|---|---|---|---|---|---|---|---|
| Brisk Walking | | | | | | | |
| Gardening | | | | | | | |
| Mowing lawn | | | | | | | |
| Stretching Exercises | | | | | | | |
| Weight Lifting | | | | | | | |
| Jogging/ Running | | | | | | | |
| Aerobics | | | | | | | |
| Bicycling | | | | | | | |
| Stair Climbing | | | | | | | |
| Swimming | | | ✓ | | | ✓ | |
| Tennis | | | | | | | |
| Bowling | | | | | | | |
| Golf | | | | | | | |
| Other Sports | | | | | | | |
| Dancing | ✓ | | | | | | |
| Other Activities | | | | | | | |

JANE

| ACTIVITY | Mon. | Tues. | Wed. | Thurs. | Fri. | Sat. | Sun. |
|---|---|---|---|---|---|---|---|
| Brisk Walking | ✓ | | ✓ | ✓ | | ✓ | |
| Gardening | | | ✓ | | | | |
| Mowing lawn | | | | | | | |
| Stretching Exercises | | | | | | | |
| Weight Lifting | | | | | | | |
| Jogging/ Running | | | | | | | |
| Aerobics | | | | | | | |
| Bicycling | | | | | | | |
| Stair Climbing | | | | | | | |
| Swimming | | | | | | | |
| Tennis | | | | | | | |
| Bowling | | | | | | | |
| Golf | | | | | | | |
| Other Sports | | | | | | | |
| Dancing | | | | | | | |
| Other Activities | | | | | | | |

| ACTIVITY | Mon. | Tues. | Wed. | Thurs. | Fri. | Sat. | Sun. |
|---|---|---|---|---|---|---|---|
| Brisk Walking | | | | | | | |
| Gardening | | | | | | | |
| Mowing lawn | | | | | | | |
| Stretching Exercises | | | | | | | |
| Weight Lifting | | | | | | | |
| Jogging/ Running | | | | | | | |
| Aerobics | | | | | | | |
| Bicycling | | | | | | | |
| Stair Climbing | | | | | | | |
| Swimming | | | | | | | |
| Tennis | | | | | | | |
| Bowling | | | | | | | |
| Golf | | | | | | | |
| Other Sports | | | | | | | |
| Dancing | | | | | | | |
| Other Activities | | | | | | | |

- old age

- cigarette smoking

- stress

- poor nutrition

- fatigue and lack of sleep

- overtraining

More and more research is finding a link between moderate, regular exercise and a strong immune system. Early studies reported that recreational exercisers report fewer colds once they began running. More recent studies have shown that there are physiological changes in the immune system response to exercise.

During moderate exercise immune cells circulate through the body more quickly, and are better able to kill bacteria and viruses. After the exercise ends the immune system returns to normal within a few hours. However consistent regular exercise seems to make these changes a bit more long-lasting. According to professor David Nieman of Appalachian State University, when moderate exercise is repeated on a near-daily basis there is a cumulative effect that leads to a long-term immune response. His research showed that those who walk at 70 to 75 per cent of their maximum heart rate for forty minutes per day had half as many sick days due to colds or sore throats as those who don't exercise.

We hope that you are convinced enough to make at least the most moderate start to improving your fitness level by means of an exercise programme. In order to help you here is a sample exercise chart that you can use to plan your programme. It will also serve as a very valuable reminder of the progress you are making in not only recovering from a mood disorder, but becoming in the process healthier and fitter than you were before. We are also including some sample charts that had been filled in so that you get a good start in understanding what is required. Remember, whatever your preferred exercise whether it be leisurely walking in a safe local park, jogging, dancing, cycling or perhaps joining your local gym, it is virtually impossible for you not to feel better as a result and to enjoy the benefits of improved mood. On our three sample patients that we described in Chapter 1, they all began or resumed some programme of exercise. Tony joined a gym near his office, Jane resumed her ballroom dancing activities and Susan took up both walking and jogging, joining both a local walking and a jogging group in the process to give her guidance and encouragement. All three were extremely happy and enthusiastic as a result.

## NUTRITION

With exercise of course goes nutrition, the other half of the equation that is the very foundation of good health and a long and happy life. There are a number of aspects of nutrition that need to be examined to be sure that your diet is optimum for you. Are you eating foods to which you have some kind of an intolerance or allergy? What kind of balance should you maintain between carbohydrates, proteins and fats? How important is fresh food in maintaining an adequate diet. And once these basic nutrition questions have been answered in such a way that best suits the type of person you are, the huge question mark is are there any foods that play an important role in helping to maintain a good balanced mood and avoid or mitigate mood disorders? We feel that there most definitely.

Initially let's consider your basic nutritional needs. Developing healthy eating habits isn't as confusing or as restrictive as many people imagine. The first principle of a healthy diet is simply to eat a wide variety of foods. This is important because different foods make different nutritional contributions.

Secondly, fruits, vegetables, grains, and legume (foods high in complex carbohydrates, fibre, vitamins, and minerals, low in fat, and free of cholesterol) should make up the bulk of the calories you consume. The rest should come from low fat dairy products, lean meat and poultry, and fish.

You should also try to maintain a balance between calorie intake and calorie expenditure. That is, do not eat more food than your body can utilise. Otherwise, you will gain weight. The more active you are therefore, the more you can eat and still maintain this balance.

Following these three basic steps does not mean you have to give up your favorite foods. As long as your overall diet is balanced and rich in nutrients and fibre, there is nothing wrong with an occasional cheeseburger. Just be sure to limit how frequently you eat such foods, and try to eat small portions of them.

You can also view healthy eating as an opportunity to expand your range of choices by trying foods—especially vegetables, whole grains, or fruits—that you don't normally eat. A healthy diet doesn't have to mean eating foods that are bland or unappealing.

The following basic guidelines are what you need to know to construct a healthy diet.

- Eat plenty of vitamins, minerals and phytochemicals (plant chemicals essential to good health).

- Make sure to include green, orange and yellow fruits and vegetables—such as broccoli, carrots, cantaloupe and citrus fruits. The antioxidants and other nutrients in these foods may help protect against developing certain types of cancer and other diseases. Eat five or more servings a day.

- Limit your intake of sugary foods, refined-grain products such as white bread and salty snack foods. Sugar, our number one additive, is added to a vast array of foods. Just one daily can of cola can add up to a considerable amount of sugar intake over the course of a year. Many sugary foods are also high in fat, so they are very high in calories.

- Cut down on animal fat. It's rich in saturated fat, which boosts blood cholesterol levels and has other adverse health effects. Choose lean meats, skinless poultry and non or low-fat dairy products.

- Cut down on trans fats, supplied by hydrogenated vegetable oils used in most processed foods in the supermarket and in many fast foods.

- Eat more fish and nuts, which contain healthy unsaturated fats. Substitute olive or canola oil for butter or margarine.

- Keep portions moderate, especially of high calorie foods. In recent years serving sizes have ballooned, particularly in restaurants. Choose a starter instead of an entrée, split a dish with a friend and do not order supersized anything.

- Keep your cholesterol intake below 300 milligrams per day. Cholesterol is found only in animal products, such as meats, poultry, dairy products and egg yolks.

- Eat a variety of foods. Do not try to fill your nutrient requirements by eating the same foods day in, day out. It is possible that not every essential nutrient has been identified, and so eating a wide assortment of foods helps to ensure that you will get all the necessary nutrients. In addition, this will limit your exposure to any pesticides or toxic substances that may be present in one particular food.

- Maintain an adequate calcium intake. Calcium is essential for strong bones and teeth. Get your calcium from low-fat sources, such as skimmed milk and low-fat yogurt. If you can't get the optimal amount from foods, take supplements.

- Try to get your vitamins and minerals from foods, not from supplements. Supplements cannot substitute for a healthy diet, which supplies nutrients and other compounds besides vitamins and minerals. Foods also provide the "synergy" that many nutrients require to be efficiently used in the body.

- Maintain a desirable weight. Balance energy (calorie) intake with energy output. Exercise and other physical activity are essential.

- If you drink alcohol, do so in moderation. Excess alcohol consumption leads to a variety of health problems. Alcoholic can add many calories to your diet without supplying nutrients. Eat plenty of high fibre foods such as fruit, vegetables, beans and whole grains. These are the "good" carbohydrates—nutritious, filling and relatively low in calories. They should supply the twenty to thirty grams of dietary fibre you need every day. This slows the absorption of carbohydrates, so there's less effect on insulin and blood sugar, and provides other health benefits as well. Such foods also provide important vitamins.

These are simple steps that you can work towards to modify your diet and nutrition so that in combination with even the most modest exercise programme it is virtually guaranteed to lift your mood in any given situation. However, the next question we will consider, are there foods that can be helpful in lifting mood?

If you do not feel good about yourself, and don't have someone supportive to listen to, this can be a major cause of lower or altered state of mood, however good your diet might be. There are a number of nutritional imbalances that can make you prone to poor mood, anxiety and depression. These are:

- essential fats – do you need more Omega 3?

- your homocysteine level – is it too high, corrected with B vitamins?

- serotonin levels – do they need boosting with amino acids?

- blood sugar balance – is yours within the healthy range?

- Chromium – are you getting enough?

So here are some suggestions to get you started with some of these foods, vitamins and minerals. This list is by no means definitive and you would be well advised to explore online sites to find out yourself how other people are reporting benefits from other foods of this type.

## INCREASE YOUR OMEGA 3 FATS

The richest dietary source is from fish, specifically carnivorous cold water fish, such as salmon, mackerel and herring. Surveys have shown that the more fish a country eats the lower is their incidence of depression. There's a type of omega 3 fat called EPA which seems to be the most potent natural anti-depressant. Again, let's examine the evidence.

There have been six double-blind placebo controlled trials to date, five of which show significant improvement. The first trial by Dr Andrew Stoll from Harvard Medical School, published in the Archives of General Psychiatry, gave forty depressed patients either omega 3 supplements versus placebo and found a highly significant improvement. The next, published in the American Journal of Psychiatry, tested the effects of giving twenty people suffering from severe depression, who were already on anti-depressants but still depressed, a highly concentrated form of omega 3 fat, called ethyl-EPA versus a placebo. By the third week the depressed patients were showing major improvement in their mood, while those on placebo were not. The latest trial by Dr Sophia

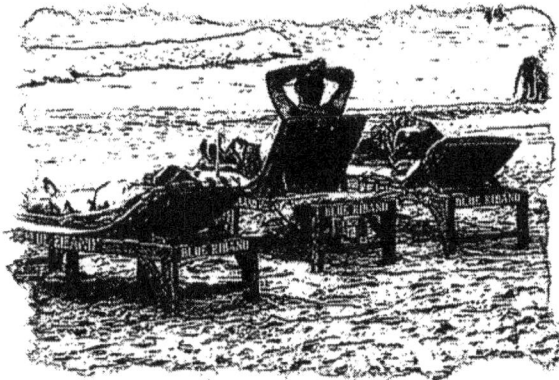

Frangou from the Institute of Psychiatry in London gave a concentrated form of EPA, versus placebo, to twenty six depressed people with bipolar disorder (manic depression) and again found a significant improvement. Of those that measured the Hamilton Rating Scale, including one recent 'open' trial not involving placebos, published last year the average improvement in depression was approximately double that shown by anti-depressant drugs, without the side-effects. This may be because omega 3s help to build your brain's neuronal connections as well as the receptor sites for neurotransmitters. Therefore the more omega-3s in your blood, the more serotonin you are likely to make and the more responsive you become to its effects.

**SIDE EFFECTS?**

In some earlier studies which gave fourteen fish oil capsules a day mild gastrointestinal discomfort, mainly loose bowels. However, nowadays you can buy more concentrated EPA rich fish oils so the amount of actual fish oil required is less. Supplementing fish oils also reduces risk for heart disease, reduces arthritic pain and may improve memory and concentration.

## INCREASE YOUR INTAKE OF B VITAMINS

People with either low blood levels of the B-vitamin folic acid, or high blood levels of the protein homocysteine, (a sign that you are not getting enough B6, B12 or folic acid) are both more likely to be depressed and less likely to get a positive result from anti-depressant drugs. In a study comparing the effects of giving an SSRI with either a placebo or with folic acid, 61% of patients improved on the placebo combination but 93% improved with the addition of folic acid. But how does folic acid itself, a cheap vitamin with no known side-effects, compare to anti-depressants?

Three trials involving 247 people addressed this question. Two involving 151 people assessed the use of folic acid in addition to other treatment, and found that adding folic acid reduced HRS scores on average by a further 2.65 points. That's not as good as the results with 5-HTP but as good, if not better than antidepressants. These studies also show that more patients treated with folate experienced a reduction in their Hamilton Rating score of greater than 50% after ten weeks compared to those on anti-depressants.

Having a high level of homocysteine, a toxic protein found in the blood, doubles the odds of a woman developing depression. The ideal level is below 6, and certainly below 9. The average level is 10-11. Depression risk doubles with levels above 15. The higher your level the more likely folic acid will work for you.

Folic acid is one of seven nutrients – the others being B2, B6, B12, zinc, magnesium and TMG – that help normalise homocysteine. Deficiency in vitamin B3, B6, folic acid, zinc and magnesium have all been linked to depression. Having a low intake of these nutrients means your brain is good at 'methylating' which is the process by which the brain keeps it's chemistry in balance. So it makes sense to both eat wholefoods, fruits, vegetables, nuts and seeds, which are high in these nutrients and supplementing a multivitamin.

**SIDE EFFECTS?**

There are none, except lower risk for heart disease, strokes, Alzheimer's Disease and improved energy and concentration. However, if you are vegan and B12 deficient, taking folic acid on its own can mask the symptoms, but the underlying nerve damage caused by B12 deficiency anaemia can persist. So, don't take folic acid without also supplementing vitamin B12.

## BOOST YOUR SEROTONIN WITH AMINO ACIDS

Serotonin is made in the body and brain from an amino acid 5-Hydroxy Tryptophan (5-HTP), which in turn is made from another amino acid called Tryptophan. Both can be found in the diet. Tryptophan is in many protein rich foods such as meat, fish, beans and eggs, while the richest source of 5-HTP is the African Griffonia bean. Just not getting enough tryptophan is likely to make you depressed.

Both have been shown to have an antidepressant effect in clinical trials, although 5HTP is more effective - 27 studies, involving 990 people to date, most of which proved effective. . So how do they compare with anti-depressants? In play-off studies between 5-HTP and SSRI antidepressants, 5-HTP generally comes out slightly better. One double-blind trial headed by Dr. Poldinger at the Basel University of Psychiatry gave 34 depressed volunteers either the SSRI fluvoxamine (Luvox) or 300 mg of 5-HTP. At the end of the six weeks, both groups of patients had had a significant improvement in their depression. However, those taking 5-HTP had a slightly greater improvement, compared to those on the SSRI, in each of the four criteria assessed—depression, anxiety, insomnia, and physical symptoms—as well as the their own self-assessment, although this improvement was not statistically significant.

Anti-depressant drugs in some sensitive people can induce an overload of serotonin called 'serotonin syndrome' characterised by feeling hot, high blood pressure, twitching, cramping, dizziness and disorientation. Some concern has been expressed about the possibility of increasing the odds of serotonin syndrome with the combination of 5-HTP and an SSRI drug. However a recent review on the safety of 5-HTP concludes that 'serotonin syndrome has not been reported in humans in association with 5-HTP, either as monotherapy (on its own) or in combination with other medications.'

Exercise, sunlight and reducing your stress level also tend to promote serotonin.

### SIDE-EFFECTS?

Some people experience mild gastrointestinal disturbance on 5-HTP, which usually stops within a few days. Since there are serotonin receptors in the gut, which don't normally expect to get the real thing so easily, they can overreact if the amount is too high resulting in transient nausea. If so, just lower the dose.

## BALANCE YOUR BLOOD SUGAR

There is a direct link between mood and blood sugar balance. All carbohydrate foods are broken down into glucose and your brain runs on glucose. The more uneven your blood sugar supply the more uneven your mood.

- Eating lots of sugar is going to give you sudden peaks and troughs in the amount of glucose in your blood. Symptoms include fatigue, irritability, dizziness, insomnia, excessive sweating (especially at night), poor concentration and forgetfulness, excessive thirst, depression and crying spells, digestive disturbances and blurred vision. Since the brain depends on an even supply of glucose it is no surprise that sugar has been implicated in aggressive behaviour, anxiety, depression and fatigue.

- Lots of refined sugar and refined carbohydrates (white bread, pasta, rice and most processed foods,) is also linked with depression because these foods not only supply very little in the way of nutrients but they also use up the mood enhancing B vitamins. Sugar also diverts the supply of another nutrient we haven't mentioned yet but is also involved in mood – Chromium. This mineral is vital for keeping your blood sugar level stable because insulin, which clears glucose from the blood, can't work properly without it. (see next section)

- The best way to keep your blood sugar level even is to eat what is called a low Glycaemic Load (GL) diet and avoid, as much as you can, refined sugar and refined foods. Instead eat whole foods, fruit, vegetables and regular meals. The book, the Holford Low GL Diet, explains exactly how to do this. Caffeine also has a direct effect on your blood sugar and your mood and is best kept to a minimum, as is alcohol.

**SIDE EFFECTS?**

None.

**INCREASE INTAKE OF CHROMIUM**

This mineral is vital for keeping your blood sugar level stable because insulin, which clears glucose from the blood, can't work properly without it. In fact just supplying proper levels of Chromium to certain depressed patients can make a big difference.

If you answer yes to a five or more of these questions you may be suffering from what's called "atypical" depression.

- Do you crave sweets or other carbohydrates?

- Do you tend to gain weight?

- Are you tired for no obvious reason?

- Do your arms or legs feel heavy?

- Do you tend to feel sleepy or groggy much of the time?

- Are your feelings easily hurt by the rejection of others?

- Did your depression begin before the age of 30?

It is called atypical because in 'classic' depression people lose their appetite, don't eat enough, lose weight and can't sleep. It affects between 25 to 42 percent of the depressed population, and an even higher percentage among depressed women, so it is extremely common rather than 'atypical'. A chance discovery by Dr Malcolm McLeod, clinical professor of psychiatry at the University of North Carolina, suggested that people who suffer with 'atypical' depression might benefit from chromium supplementation.

In a small double-blind study McLeod gave ten patients suffering from atypical depression Chromium supplements of 600mcg a-day and five others a placebo for eight weeks. The results were dramatic. Seven out of ten taking the supplements showed a big improvement, versus none on the placebo. Their Hamilton Rating Score for depression dropped by an unheard of 83%; from 29 - major depression - to 5 – not depressed. A larger trial at Cornell University with 113 patients has confirmed the finding. After eight weeks 65% of those on Chromium had had a major improvement, compared to 33% on placebos.

**SIDE EFFECTS?**

None, except more energy and better weight control. Chromium, if taken in the evening, can increase energy and hence interfere with sleep. Chromium has no toxicity even at amounts 100 times this.

At the end of Chapter 6 your task is to print out or exercise and nutrition charts of the examples through this chapter and begin planning your own programme of improved nutrition and exercise. You must take it slowly, at least to begin with. If you try to rush into a heavy exercise programme the end result will either be the opposite of what you are trying to achieve-you could find that your mood is lowered rather than the opposite because of the excessive demands you put on your body. In a similar way with a diet and possibly supplement programme a sudden change of diet could upset your system and metabolism so again it has the opposite effect from what you are seeking i.e. you experience a lowered mood rather than an increased feeling of well-being. A slow and gentle approach will give your body and mind time to adjust and really reap the benefits of the positive changes you are making to it.

## TASKS

- Please fill in a mood loss and nutrition chart and keep it with the other
- Please fill in a further mood compass when you are done with the mood loss and nutrition charts.

*Nothing lifts me out of a bad mood better than a hard workout on my treadmill. It never fails. To us, exercise is nothing short of a miracle.*

*Cher*

EXERCISE

| Nutrition Journal | Sunday | | Monday | | Tuesday | | Wednesday | | Thursday | | Friday | | Saturday | |
|---|---|---|---|---|---|---|---|---|---|---|---|---|---|---|
| | Cals | Fat Grams | Cals | Fat Grams | Cals | Fat Grams | Cals | Fat Grams | Cals | Fat Grams | Cals | Fat Grams | Cals | Fat Grams |
| Meal One | | Time | | Time | | Time | | Time | | Time | | Time | | Time |
| Meal Two | | Time | | Time | | Time | | Time | | Time | | Time | | Time |
| Meal Three | | Time | | Time | | Time | | Time | | Time | | Time | | Time |
| Meal Four | | Time | | Time | | Time | | Time | | Time | | Time | | Time |
| Meal Five | | Time | | Time | | Time | | Time | | Time | | Time | | Time |
| Total | | Time | | Time | | Time | | Time | | Time | | Time | | Time |

97

| Day | Date | Weight (lbs) |
|-----|------|--------------|
| 42 | | |
| 43 | | |
| 44 | | |
| 45 | | |
| 46 | | |
| 47 | | |
| 48 | | |
| 49 | | |
| 50 | | |
| 51 | | |
| 52 | | |
| 53 | | |
| 54 | | |
| 55 | | |
| 56 | | |
| 57 | | |
| 58 | | |
| 59 | | |
| 60 | | |
| 61 | | |
| 62 | | |

| Day | Date | Weight (lbs) |
|-----|------|--------------|
| 21 | | |
| 22 | | |
| 23 | | |
| 24 | | |
| 25 | | |
| 26 | | |
| 27 | | |
| 28 | | |
| 29 | | |
| 30 | | |
| 31 | | |
| 32 | | |
| 33 | | |
| 34 | | |
| 35 | | |
| 36 | | |
| 37 | | |
| 38 | | |
| 39 | | |
| 40 | | |
| 41 | | |

| Day | Date | Weight (lbs) |
|-----|------|--------------|
| 0 | | |
| 1 | | |
| 2 | | |
| 3 | | |
| 4 | | |
| 5 | | |
| 6 | | |
| 7 | | |
| 8 | | |
| 9 | | |
| 10 | | |
| 11 | | |
| 12 | | |
| 13 | | |
| 14 | | |
| 15 | | |
| 16 | | |
| 17 | | |
| 18 | | |
| 19 | | |
| 20 | | |

EXERCISE

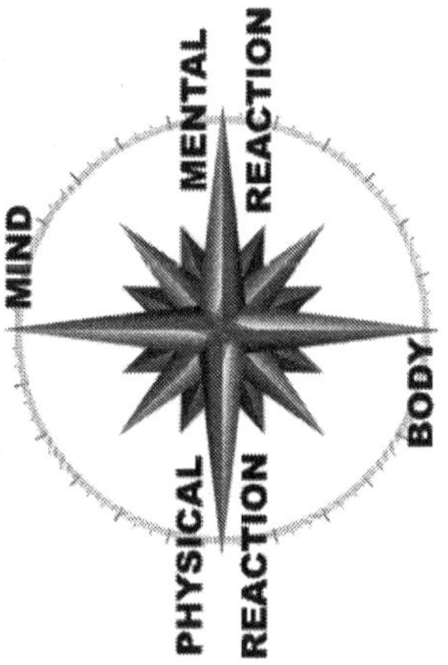

This part of the book introduces some of the key concepts such as the Mind Compass and helps you to understand some of the underlying causes of various moods. Several cases are examined and at the end of the chapter you will find a list of useful exercises to carry out to help reinforce your learning.

# CHAPTER 7: SITUATIONS

# CHAPTER 7: SITUATIONS

*The secret of man's success resides in his insight into the mood's of people, and his tact in dealing with them.*

*Josiah Gilbert Holland*

It will be clear by now that one of the major difficulties experienced by low mood sufferers is in misunderstanding situations. and interpreting them in an unhelpful and inappropriate negative fashion, when a positive interpretation would be more helpful. There is no doubt that sufferers of lowered and negative mood conditions and see themselves in a different way than non-sufferers do. For example, low mood it brings about such feelings as:

- i'm not a good person

- i totally failed to carry out the task

- i'll never learn to do this

- the last couple of months have gone really badly for me

- that's me, I always get the rough end of the deal

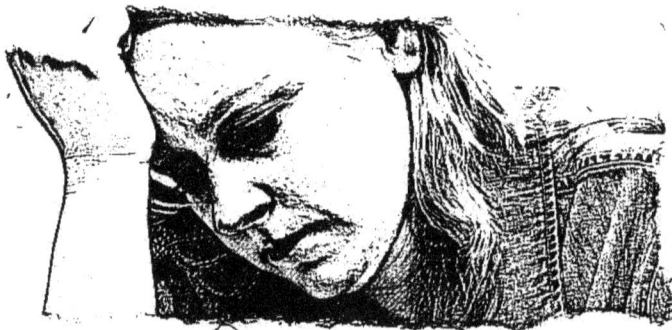

These are the kinds of thoughts that you may recall popping into your head at different times. Surely it will come as no surprise to you to understand that the more often you think in this way, the more it will become a self-perpetuating prophecy. We hope that you have started to make regular use of the charts that we have introduced to you to keep a record of your moods and thinking, so that you can challenge the very perceptions that you have of yourself, of other people and of situations so that you can see them in a much more positive and realistic light.

# SITUATIONS

As a simple rule of thumb you could take a simple three-step approach to dealing with thoughts that you know are unhelpful to you. If you want something to help you remember this process, remember the three point turn that is a part of the driving test. (In fact these days there can be more than three points taken to turn a car around, but in this exercise lets keep the fabled three-point turn as our memory marker.) The three-point turn analogy has not been chosen at random, for the object of this turn is to turn the car around and pointed in the opposite direction. Your simple three-step approach, your "three-point turn" is used in an almost identical way, to turn your thoughts around and point them in the opposite direction. From negative to positive, from bad to good, from miserable to happy, from unhelpful to helpful. Remember the three point turn, it goes like this:

- Firstly single out the uncomfortable and unhelpful thought you had, put it into words, write it down if possible although this is not essential.

- Be honest with yourself and ask yourself a simple question. Did this thought help you in any way or was it really unhelpful, at the very least to your mood and general mind state?

- Now for the important part. What kind of thought would have been helpful and comfortable to you?

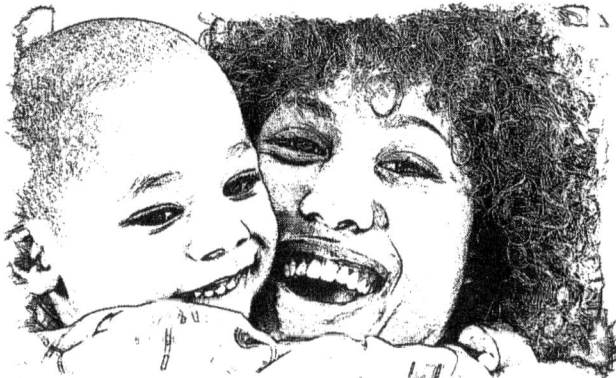

The questioning process is important to enable you to recognise the ways in which you are self inflicting damage upon yourself, totally unnecessarily. It also allows you to embark on a process of changing and balancing your thinking in such a way that you will get to the point where more comfortable, balanced and helpful thinking and mental reactions to different events will occur to you automatically.

Let's take a look at an example. This patient's name was Julie, a 24 year old woman, a single parent with a five year old son.

She was concerned that she was finding it extremely difficult to cope with looking after a young child, holding down a responsible job (she was the manager of a local ladies fashion shop) and juggling with the inevitable financial overload that is the lot of so many single parents. Lately she had begun to find

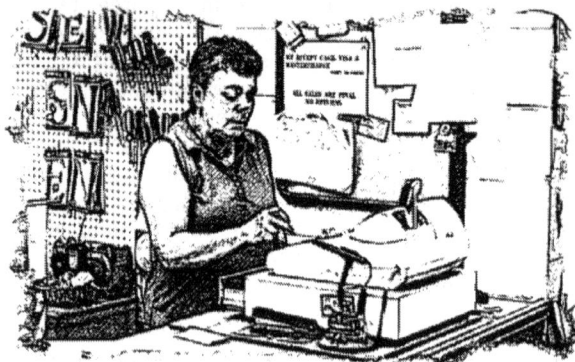

herself snapping at customers and staff in the shop, to the extent that her area manager had taken her quietly to one side and asked her if she had a problem. Fortunately the area manager was sympathetic and chatted to Julie about her feelings. It was at this stage that she came to us to discuss the way she was feeling and what she could do about it. It soon became apparent that Julie was suffering from symptoms of anxiety and slight depression. She told us the story of an event that happened recently in her shop. A customer came into the store looking for a particular type of outfit, a skirt with a matching top. The lady was fairly elderly and it took Julie every ounce of her patience to show the lady what was available and comment on the outfit as she tried them on. The woman seemed very unappreciative of the extreme lengths to which Julie was going to help her out and eventually Julie considered that the woman was downright rude. Nonetheless, she was elderly and Julie managed to get through the session and make the sale. By the time the woman left the store Julie felt that the woman's rudeness had been almost abusive and she was very angry both at the customer and at herself for not having dealt with the situation in a better way. She felt somehow diminished, that she had demonstrated an approach to her job that was less than professional and was even angry at herself for feeling so bad about such a situation.

The following day a young woman came into the store. She described the elderly woman that Julie had served the day before and explained that she was the woman's daughter. She was absolutely delighted with the patient help that Julie had given to her mother and said that the outfit looked extremely nice. The mother had recently been widowed and had been unable to leave the house for several months, having been diagnosed with anxiety and depression symptoms. Julie's patient help had gone a long way towards restoring her confidence. Apparently she had been dreading going shopping for a new outfit and was extremely pleased that the outcome was so successful. It need hardly be added that this was the strongest possible message to Julie that her understanding of a given situation or event had taken the most negative and unhelpful perception possible. Working in retail shops must be very difficult at times but the prospect of an elderly customer being recently widowed, or perhaps another could be recovering from a serious illness is hardly an uncommon scenario. Julie was able to see that the most negative interpretation or perception of an event was invariably going to be incorrect and not only that extremely unhelpful to her.

Are we talking about transforming our thinking from negative to positive here? Well, yes we are, at least in a way. Quite apart from interpretation and perception, there are other factors that are in play when we view things in a certain way. Whether you are a positive or a negative thinker, it is interesting to find out the chemical and physical changes that occur within the body. Many fail to realise that both negative and positive thinking can trigger chemical and physical changes within the body. There are a multitude of benefits that extend beyond positive thinking, just as there are many downsides associated with negative thinking. Positive thinking is known for its numerous benefits on overall health. Negative thinking is known for its detrimental effects on overall health and well being. And even though change can occur in a number of different ways for different thoughts, these changes can alter the way that one responds to the environment and vice versa.

When positive thinking occurs, people have better back posture, their thoughts are clearer and concise, and there's a good feeling within the self which allows them to accomplish many tasks. By being able to change thoughts from negative to positive one can develop a sense of self-confidence, which gives the ability to tackle challenges head-on. These chemical and physical changes can have a significant affect on one's overall health.

Chemical and physical changes within the body can include:

- release of endorphins within the brain
- relaxed state of mind
- ability to think more clearly
- more likely to make rational decisions
- good amount of self-confidence
- good back posture

Negative thinking can also trigger an array of chemical and physical changes within the body, including:

- decreased flow of endorphins
- poor back posture
- lack of self-confidence
- cluttered mind
- racing thoughts
- increased likelihood of making irrational decision - poor judgment

People tend to avoid people who are consistently negative. A lot can be learned by body language alone. Even when a person does not speak, people can feel negative vibes from a person who does not have a positive demeanor. According to the article, "Hardwired for Happiness", written by The Dana Foundation in the 1990s, Antonio Damasio, M.D., Ph.D., discovered that positive and negative feelings are both generated and processed by different parts of the human brain.

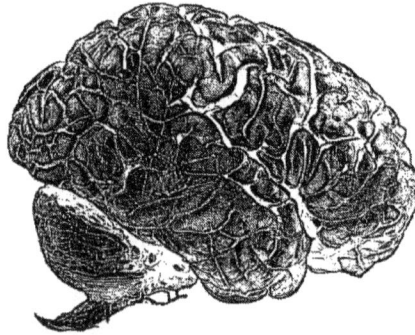

Numerous studies have shown the benefits of being able to change thoughts from negative to positive. Many of these studies have shown that endorphins within the brain (also known as feel good chemicals that help balance mood) are actually hindered when negative thinking patterns are in effect. Over time these thinking behaviors have a detrimental affect on overall health.

Many studies have associated the anterior cingulate cortex with the regulation of emotions, so it has been named "the affective division" of the cingulate cortex. It also appears to be altered in people with depression, for whom happiness is difficult to achieve.

Positive thinking, on the other hand, provides a good boost of endorphins within the brain and allows people to have a feeling of contentment within the self and a good amount of confidence. These chemical and physical changes help to create a well balanced individual with optimal mental and physical well being. These chemical and physical changes also have positive effects on the body's physical composition. Have you ever noticed a person that exemplifies confidence? They have good back posture, a positive attitude and people tend to be drawn to them.

During the depths of her suffering Jane frequently snapped at her husband, who she thought was being overly critical of the way she was spending so much time at home and away from her regular activities. On one occasion the arguments became so intense that Jane began wondering did he have some sort of alternative motive for wanting her out of the house. Could it be that late in life he had taken a lover and was trying to get her out of the house so that the coast would be clear? Was there some other reason? Did her husband just not like, did he not enjoy her company and not want her around? It was clear to her that something was amiss with her husband and on one occasion she did decide to go back to her dancing class to in effect test out her theories.

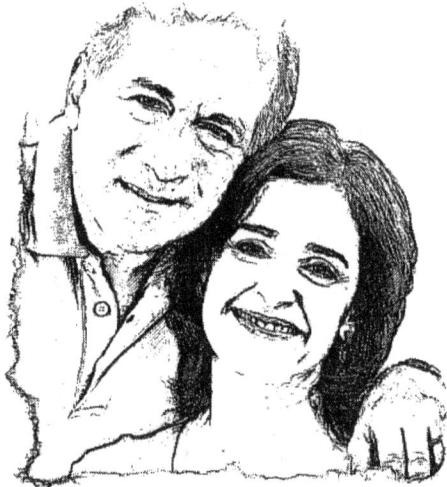

The dancing class is itself was unsuccessful, for some reason however friends, or at least those women who used to be her friends, were not able to understand the difficulties she was having. For some reason they seemed less than interested in hearing about her problems in looking after a sick husband and seemed to be making light of it. They even laughed when she told them of her suspicions about her husband. When she finally got home she was experiencing one of the blackest, lowest moods she had ever known. Did her husband just despise their, or was he seeing another woman? And what was the problem with the ladies at the dancing class? They seemed to be off with her, unsympathetic and disinclined to be receptive to hearing about any of her problems? Perhaps they were blaming her for not having attended the classes for so long. What she being frozen out?

## MOOD CHECK CHART

During her therapy, we gave Jane a mood check chart. This is a very simple device, and allows the sufferer to at least form an assessment of whether there thinking is helpful or unhelpful to them.

Here is an example:

MOOD CHECK CHART

- Do you feel downhearted, blue and sad?
- Do you feel worse in the morning?
- Do you have crying spells, or feel like it?
- Do you have trouble falling asleep, or sleeping through the night?
- Is your appetite poor?
- Are you losing weight without trying?
- Do you feel unattractive and unlovable?
- Do you prefer to be alone?
- Do you feel fearful?
- Are you often tired and irritable?
- Is it an effort to do the things you used to do?
- Are you restless and unable to keep still?
- Do you feel hopeless about the future?
- Do you find it difficult to make decisions?
- Do you feel less enjoyment from activities that once gave you pleasure?

If you answered yes to:

**Less than 5:** You are normal. You appear to be positive, optimistic and able to roll with the punches. The information below will give you clues on how to handle those occasions when things aren't going so well for you.

107

**5 to 10:** You have a mild to moderate case of the blues. Read on to see how this can happen, and then to the solutions. You might also consider seeking outside help.

**More than 10:** You are moderately to markedly depressed. Besides following the advice below, we recommend you seek professional help.

How do we know that a storm is about to break? Perhaps we hear thunder in the distance, the skies are dark and grey with rain clouds, and it becomes very windy. If we do not want to be caught with the worst effects of the storm, we would probably go back home, close all the windows, bring our washing in from the line and secure any loose items outside the house. Similarly, if bipolar patients become more aware of their early warning signs that signal the onset of a mood episode, they can take steps to prevent a full-blown episode of depression and mania.

Early detection of an impending "storm" - in the case of bipolar disorder, an episode of mania or depression - can lead to early intervention and prevention of a mood episode. In order to be able to detect an oncoming episode, bipolar patients must learn to recognise their own early warning signs and symptoms of their illness. Each person has their own unique set of signs and symptoms although many will be common to other patients.

It is not enough to be able to recognise and detect early warning signs and symptoms of a mood episode. You need also to monitor them regularly. It will not be much good if you are aware of your early warning signs and symptoms, but you continue to go through your daily life without paying much attention to the onset of the symptoms. Similarly, a person who knows that ominous grey clouds, thunder, lightning, and rushing wind signal an impending storm can still get caught in the storm if they were sitting on a park bench too engrossed in a book to look around them. Therefore, regular self monitoring is important for the purpose of early intervention to prevent relapse.

The first step to self monitoring is monitoring your mood for the day.

Ask yourself,

- How did I feel today?

- Was my mood within the normal range, or was I feeling slightly low or high?

- How low?

- How high?

- Rate your mood, between -5 (depressed) and +5 (manic). Try to rate your mood at the same time everyday.

Try using the thought records to monitor your thoughts. Try it for a week and see if you can identify any pattern in your mood fluctuations. You might also want to take note of the circumstances in which you experienced particularly high or low moods. Bring your completed thought monitoring worksheets to your doctor or mental health professional and discuss your observations with them, if you so wish.   Another way of monitoring yourself is to identify and be aware of any signs and symptoms associated with a low mood that you might be experiencing. If you experience a number of these symptoms over a few days, in such a way that they interfere with most of your day-to-day activities, you might want to consider taking some action. We will talk about planning early interventions a little later on.

Firstly, over the next week, monitor mood change in your daily mood by filling in the weekly chart.

Each day indicate if you have experienced any of the symptoms listed in the chart, in a way that they have interfered with most of your day-to-day activities. You might also want to record any observations you may have about the circumstances in which you experienced these symptoms.

### WEEKLY MOOD CHANGE CHART

|  | Day 1 | Day 2 | Day 3 | Day 4 | Day 5 | Day 6 | Day 7 |
|---|---|---|---|---|---|---|---|
| Date: | | | | | | | |
| Loss of interest or pleasure | | | | | | | |
| Increase or decrease in appetite | | | | | | | |
| Unable to sleep or sleep too much | | | | | | | |
| Physically agitated or slowed down | | | | | | | |
| Fatigue or loss of energy | | | | | | | |
| Feeling worthless or guilty | | | | | | | |
| Unable to concentrate or make decisions | | | | | | | |
| Thoughts of death or suicide | | | | | | | |
| Elevated or irritable mood | | | | | | | |
| Increased self-esteem or self-confidence | | | | | | | |
| Decreased need for sleep | | | | | | | |
| More talkative than usual | | | | | | | |
| Racing thoughts | | | | | | | |
| Easily distracted | | | | | | | |
| Increase in goal-directed activity | | | | | | | |
| Overly eager in pleasurable activities | | | | | | | |

Early warning signs of a relapse or an episode recurrence are symptoms that typically signal the onset of a mood episode. Some patients may think that they are not able to predict an episode but researchers have found that many bipolar patients are able to recall early warning symptoms that come before a full-blown episode. Bipolar patients have commonly reported increased activity, decreased need for sleep, and elevated mood

It was noted that although there were some differences in the specific early warning symptoms experienced by patients, these symptoms appeared to be the same within each patient in subsequent episodes. Thus, although some early warning symptoms may be unique to individual patients, it appears that they are quite accurate in predicting the onset of a mood episode for each patient.

To identify your early warning signs of lowered mood, a finer analysis needs to be done. Ask yourself, "What am I like when my mood is mildly elevated and moderately elevated? What am I like when I am mildly depressed and moderately depressed? Use the chart to record all these symptoms. When you have written them down, reflect on the three or four most prominent early warning symptoms of mania and depression. Will you be able to recognise these symptoms when you next experience them? It might be a good idea to discuss this worksheet with your doctor or appropriate health professional.

The next step is to develop an action plan that details what you will do when you recognise the early warning signs and symptoms of a major episode. It is important to be prepared so that when the time comes, you will know what to do. Plan what you will do, what you will say, what you will ask your friends and family to do for you, etc. For example, your action plan may include a visit to your doctor when you recognise your energy level has increased and are feeling restless, or you may ask a friend to keep your credit card when you have the urge to shop for shoes, or request that a relative drop by to visit you when you stop calling them, etc. You may also want to ask your friends and family to say specific things to you to highlight the possibility that you might be becoming unwell. It's probably good to let them know the best way to say it so it doesn't offend you. Detail your early intervention plans carefully and keep them on your desk or on the refrigerator - somewhere that is easily accessible or visible - so that you can refer to them when the need arises.

- What am I like when I am mildly depressed?
- What I would do to prevent a full-blown manic episode?
- What I would do to prevent a full-blown depressive episode?
- What I would ask my friends or family to do for me?
- What I would ask my friends or family to say to me?

Research has shown that for many people, their first episode was triggered by a major life stressor. Subsequent episodes have also been linked with a stressful life event. Because of this, we also encourage you to think about this and chart the course of illness in your life by doing a Life Chart. A life chart is a diagram that illustrates the number, sequence, and duration of manic and depressive episodes, beginning from the very first episode. The purpose of drawing a life chart is for you to track and identify patterns of recurrences, early warning signs and to see if there has been anything that might have triggered the onset of an episode. As such, it is important that you include in your life chart the occurrence of significant life events and the influence of treatment, such as medication and psychotherapy.

You may find it easier to begin with the most recent episode and then work backwards. Talking with family members or consulting medical records may also be beneficial. After you have completed your life chart, take a good look at all the events you have recorded. Is there any pattern of episode recurrence? Is there anything or any event that might have triggered a mood episode? Once you become more aware of the things that affect you and your moods, you can take steps to be better prepared to deal with problems or events that come your way. The ultimate goal is for you to become your own expert in dealing with and managing your illness.

The purpose of mood-monitoring, identifying early warning signs and doing a life chart is to help you become more aware of yourself, your moods, and what is going on in your life. This being so that you can manage your illness better, make informed decisions, prevent further illness episodes and ultimately have the quality of life that you want. You may think that this makes you very focused on yourself and your illness or problems. However, by monitoring your moods and symptoms, you can be more prepared for action to prevent an episode from getting out of hand and ultimately endangering yourself. Thus, the benefits of self-monitoring far outweigh the costs.

- Regular self monitoring is important for the purpose of early intervention to prevent relapse

- Mood monitoring involves rating your mood about between once a day, asking yourself, "How did I feel today? Was my mood within the normal range, or was I feeling slightly low/ high? How low (0 to -S)? How high (0 to +S)?"

- Symptom monitoring is about identifying and being aware of any signs and symptoms associated with a depressive, manic or mixed episode that interfere with most of your day-to-day activities.

- Bipolar patients commonly report increased activity, decreased need for sleep, and elevated mood as early warning signs of mania, and depressed mood, loss of energy, loss of interest in people or activities, impaired concentration and thoughts of death as early warning signs for depression.

- Identifying your early warning signs requires you to be aware of your symptoms when your mood is mildly elevated, moderately elevated, mildly depressed, and moderately depressed.

- It is important for you to develop an early intervention plan that details your most significant early warning signs, what you would do, what you could ask your friends and family to do, and what you could ask them to say to you to warn you that you might be becoming unwell.

- Stressful life events can sometimes contribute to triggering a mood episode and it would be important to be aware of how they affect you so that you can then be better prepared to deal with them.

- Consistent and regular self-monitoring and early intervention are the keys to preventing relapse and episode recurrences.

## TASKS

- Your task at the end of Chapter 7 is to work through the process of filling in weekly mood change charts.  Go back as far as you can remember, and keep the charts handy for future reference.

- Would you also fill in a further Mood Compass and keep it with the others.  Are you noting any progress yet?

*The heart loves, but moods have no loyalty. Moods should be heard but never danced to.*

*Hugh Prather*

This part of the book discusses how details from your history can prove very important with regards to planning your future. You will learn how to record all kinds of useful information that will be of benefit in later chapters.

# CHAPTER 8: HISTORY

# CHAPTER 8: HISTORY

*Therefore, let us not despair, but instead, survey the position, consider carefully the action we must take, and then address ourselves to our common task in a mood of sober resolution and quiet confidence, without haste and without pause.*

*Arthur Henderson*

## GOING IN AT THE DEEP END-TRYING SOMETHING DIFFERENT

It is by no means unusual for low mood sufferers to have fairly fixed expectations of given situations. In fact it is these fixed, and frequently incorrect, expectations that are to blame for so many problems such as low self esteem, negative self image and its close relations anxiety and depression. In this chapter we will be examining the task of filling in charts that will help us to understand where our thoughts are in need of change and modification. So we shall list events that have happened to you, the mood reaction that has occurred as a result of your wrong thinking and then you will be asked to pencil in a more suitable reaction that you plan to happen next time the event occurs.

This little story can show how someone thought about a very serious setback in their life and how their attempts to overcome it was a story of triumph over adversity.

"This past March, a business trip brought me to Granville for the first time since I was injured. I felt an avalanche of emotions flooding over me as I drove by the entrance of the path. I parked my van in the same parking place where I parked two years ago and wept. The nightmare was returning.

Often times we have bad memories tied to specific locations. Perhaps a crisis, dispute, death, injury or illness occurred in a particular place and you have not been able to return to that location due to the bad memories that it provoked.

Every time you think of, or drive near that site, you become emotional and purposely avoid going back.

That's how it has been for me for the past two years. I have purposely steered clear of the bicycle path in Granville, Ohio. On June 13, 1998 I was crushed by a tree while riding my bicycle on this path and was paralyzed from the waist down.

This past March, a business trip brought me to Granville for the first time since I was injured. I felt an avalanche of emotions flooding over me as I drove by the entrance of the path. I parked my van in the same parking place where I parked two years ago and wept. The nightmare was returning.

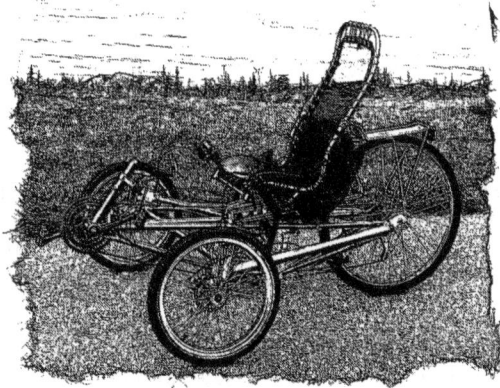

As I returned home I thought about the sense of accomplishment that I would feel if I could ride that trail again. I had been shopping for a bicycle that I would be able to pedal with my weakened legs and paralyzed feet and ankles. I had researched and tested many three wheeled recumbent style trikes and found one that met my special needs. My trike was delivered in May.

On June 13, 2000 my husband, Mark Leder, and I were off to Granville. This ride was one we both were uneasy about taking. A return to our favorite trail, yet a return to the memories of the worst day of our lives.

As we face our demons, we build courage. Courage to stand up to what we fear. For me, the act of literally standing for the first time while clenching a walker, was a courageous act. Like the properties of a magnet to repel, our bad experiences cause us to go in opposite directions to avoid a confrontation.

For so many of the tasks that I have accomplished during the past two years, I needed courage. Regaining my life back meant learning to do things all over again. It took courage to learn to drive a car with hand controls, walk with crutches, ski on a monoski and bike again.

Courage is the power to face your adversities. You are more powerful than your outside circumstances. When you recognize

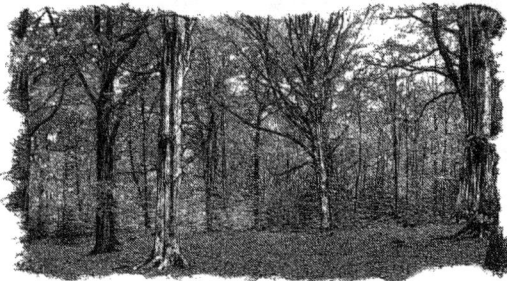

that you are bigger than your problems, you gain the courage that is necessary to overcome anything.

It is inevitable that deep emotions will come to the surface as we return to a location where sadness prevailed. A

117

purging of emotional tensions is good for spiritual healing.

Mark and I celebrated our victory over tragedy. We rode to the exact spot where the tree fell on me. We were there and the tree was gone. It was then that we were able to put many of the missing pieces together.

The site is identifiable due to the clearing in the woods where the tree once grew, the spliced electric lines, the broken branches on trees still standing, and logs cut from the tree that crushed me which lay on the side of the trail. After riding on the trail and retracing the rescue operation, we better understood how hard the rescue team worked to get me out.

It is better that we rejoice over our accomplishments following a tragedy than to dwell on self pity. What happened is in the past. It is more important that we focus on our present and future. It is as if sometimes we are dealt a hand of cards in our game of life. Sometimes the hand we are dealt is unfortunate. What we must do is to take our misfortune and make the best of it.

Many people are walking around wounded, caught up in the past and unable to make the changes that are needed to move forward. Oftentimes we disable ourselves with self limiting beliefs. We have to make some changes if we want things to change."

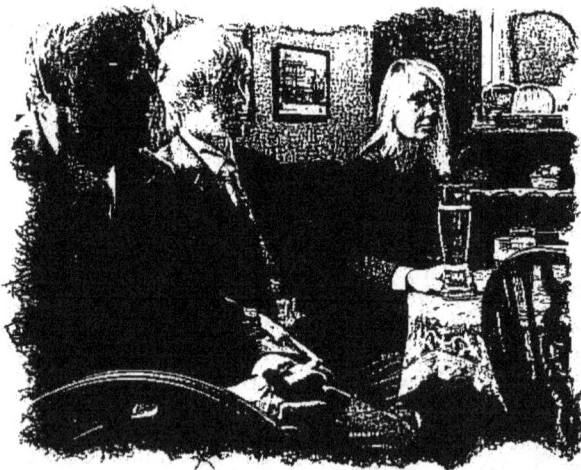

This lady had clearly experienced and extremely serious accident which left her with feelings of fear and unease. With her husband they were able to challenge this negative feeling and to experiment with a different approach. In this case re-visiting the site of the accident and finding that her perception and mood resulting from this visit was totally unlike what she had expected. Clearly she was able to turn a low mood event into a positive affair, one of triumph that left her feeling good about herself.

Tony, the cocaine addict that we discussed in Chapter 1 was invited every Friday lunchtime for drinks with his colleagues, most of whom were his juniors. He had long suspected that this invitation was rooted in some kind of malicious attempt for these colleagues to make fun of him and humiliate him in the pub. So much so that lately they had given up asking him, which he then assumed was because they were no longer interested in any kind of friendly relationship with him and viewed him effectively as an enemy. He spoke to us one week of this situation and said that quite out of the blue that they had asked him to go for the lunchtime drink last Friday. As usual he had refused. He was able to chart this on a piece of paper and could write down differing outcomes from his going for a drink with his colleagues. Of course, there was a possibility of some kind of office unpleasantness rearing its head during the lunchtime session. But on paper he had to admit that this did look slightly absurd. Other outcomes he wrote began to look more positive. That his colleagues wanted to include him in the circle of friends, if for no other reason than to oil the wheels of their working relationships. Then again, there could even be an outside possibility that one of the females in the group had taken a fancy to him and hoped that meeting him socially would advance the possibility of their attempting some sort of a relationship outside of the office. The most likely scenario was of course that these were essentially friendly decent people who included him in their invitation as a part of the accepted behaviour in the normal office environment.

We discussed this at length and eventually Tony was able to concede that the chance of a positive outcome to this social occasion was much more likely than a negative outcome. The next move was for Tony to experiment and see if by altering his attitude to these people's invitation the result could be something pleasant, something that would enhance his working relationships, rather than the negative outcome that up until now he had dwelled upon. Grasping the bull by the horns, the next day he went into the office and approached two of his colleagues directly, apologised for not having gone with them for their Friday lunchtime drink and asked them would they mind if he came along next Friday. They were obviously surprised that his approach to their weekly session had suddenly changed, but seemed genuinely pleased that he was going with them. As things turned out, he found the Friday lunchtime session to be a happy and congenial affair. One of his colleagues confided to him that they had thought that he was keeping himself aloof from them and refused to go with them because he perhaps looked at them in a rather negative way. Tony was able of course to affirm that this was the last thing on his mind, and the simple lunchtime session seemed to be the start of an improved working relationship with his colleagues and a general improvement in his mood. So what made the difference? Quite simply, Tony managed to identify an event that had been causing him some unease, was perhaps a little thorn in his side, had identified where his thinking seemed to be poorly constructed. He also identified in which ways he is negative view of the situation could have been in error and how a more positive interpretation could be much more helpful and comfortable for him. Then he took the step of putting the positive interpretation into action, in effect experimenting with a different response, one that was far more likely to be appropriate than his previous response. In this case the experiment worked well and the positive interpretation which on balance of probability was almost certainly the proper interpretation proved to be correct.

"Psychological payoff" behaviour patterns that provide some psychological rewards can also have important downsides. Common examples of these types of patterns of unwanted behavior include:

- overeating

- procrastinating

- problematic ways of interacting with other people

- excessive spending

- excessive TV or internet

We are attempting to show you how to stop unwanted behaviour patterns by understanding the hidden, and not so hidden), psychological payoffs associated with behaviour. People generally don't keep repeating behaviour patterns, unless on some level they get something good from the behaviour. Once you understand what psychological needs are entangled with the unwanted behaviour you'll be more effective at changing it and finding a more fulfilling alternative.

Let's look at the different types of payoffs that commonly draw people into patterns of unwanted behaviour.

Think about a behaviour you want to do less of. You'll get more out of reading this section if you identify one specific example from your own life and think about that example as you read. In psychologist terms, payoffs come in two varieties:

1. Getting more of something you want.

2. Experiencing less of something you don't want (avoiding difficult thoughts, numbing difficult emotions or escaping from difficult situations or tasks).

And in different domains:

- emotion payoffs

- thought payoffs

- physical payoffs

- situation payoffs

Any unwanted behaviour will have MULTIPLE different types of payoffs.

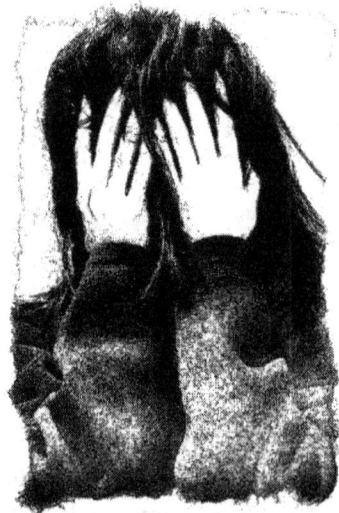

## EMOTION PAYOFFS

It is important to recognise that unwanted behaviours are often associated with a mixture of wanted and unwanted consequences. For example, when you break a diet and overeat you might feel guilt or shame, but you might also feel elements of excitement that you are rebelling against your self imposed rules. What we are trying to do here is build a full picture of all the different types of consequences of an unwanted behaviour, so that you can understand it psychologically. Does the behavior you want to do less of provide any positive emotions? Which ones?

e.g. calmness/soothing/relaxation, joy, excitement, interest.

Does this behaviour reduce your negative emotions? Which ones? e.g. anxiety/fear/tension, shame, anger, loneliness, sadness, guilt?

Sometimes emotion payoffs will only be very mild (e.g. provide a mild sense of interest or excitement, or decreasing your anger only a little bit), but include these mild payoffs in your analysis because they're part of the psychological picture. One of the most important payoffs often associated with unwanted

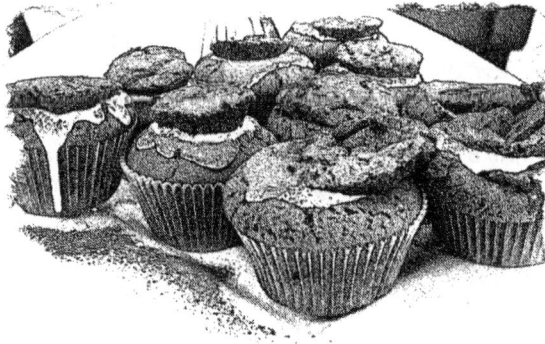

behaviour is reduced anxiety or tension. Lots of different types of unwanted behaviour help people temporarily reduce feelings of anxiety.

### THOUGHT PAYOFFS

Thought payoffs come in lots of different types. We are able to give some examples of a few of the important types here.

1. 1. Thought payoffs can include distracting yourself from thinking about something that is difficult to think about. For example, numbing yourself with media can be an effective distraction from thinking about aspects of your life and relationships.

2. 2. Another important type of thought payoff is asserting your sense of being the master of your own destiny e.g. "I'm an adult and I can do what I want". This often applies to unwanted behaviours that involve breaking your own or

other people's rules (e.g. spending money that's not in your budget or breaking a diet).

3.  3. Another important type of thought payoff relates to how you see yourself as a person and how others see you. Let's say it is really important to you that other people know you're a nice, fair, generous or fun person. If that is important to you it will be a powerful motivator of your behaviour. For example, if you view spending money freely as part of your fun-loving/carefree persona this might lead to you spending more money than you can afford. Or, wanting to be perceived as nice might lead you to be too generous in helping others. If doing an unwanted behaviour validates your sense that you're nice, fair, generous, fun (or whatever it is that's important to you), then add it to your analysis. It's an important psychological payoff. It can work the other way too, e.g. if you want other people to see you as very in control/very independent, this might interfere with getting close to people (e.g. if the unwanted behaviour you want to overcome is difficulties with relationship closeness).

4.  4. Yet another common type of thought payoff relates to "deservingness" thoughts. This is when doing the unwanted behaviour validates that you "deserve" the good outcomes that come with the unwanted behaviour. You deserve to have the thrill of buying nice things, you deserve to treat yourself, you deserve to relax. Deservingness payoffs are often particularly powerful motivators of behaviour, if underneath you are ambivalent about your deservingness or you perceive yourself as having low worth (low self esteem). One of the solutions to this is to become more comfortable that you do deserve to have your deep psychological needs.

5.  5. You can learn more about understanding your deep psychological needs here

### SURFACE VS. DEEP GOALS

Ask yourself if any of those deep needs are entangled with your unwanted behaviour.

### PHYSICAL PAYOFFS

Some types of unwanted behaviour have physical payoffs. For example for the short period after you eat a high sugar snack might have a big payoff of increased energy and reduced tiredness.

This intense short term physical payoff is likely to be very powerful in keeping you doing that unwanted behaviour during times you are tired.

## SITUATION PAYOFFS

What happens after you do the unwanted behaviour?

For example, shouting at your child or partner might be effective in making them to do what you need in the short term (even it's not helpful for those relationships in the long term).

If you shout at your partner does she/he stop nagging you?

If you smack you children, do they stop vying for your attention and give you a break? In these cases, those outcomes are part of what keeps you doing the unwanted behaviour.

Does doing the unwanted behaviour (at least temporarily) "get you out of" something you do not want to do or something that would be difficult to do?

Does sabotaging your relationships mean you avoid relationship closeness and commitment issues that would be difficult for you?

Does procrastinating at work mean you are less likely to be promoted? Do you feel ambivalent about aspects of what being promoted would mean (e.g. you don't want to do public speaking or travel, you like being one of the guys rather than a boss)?

Once you know what psychological needs are entangled with your unwanted behaviour, think more about these alternative coping strategies. These might be alternative strategies for the times when you might otherwise do the unwanted behaviour. Or, depending on what behaviour you are focusing on, they might be alternative problem solving ideas (e.g. how you could become more comfortable with relationship closeness/trust) or broader ideas about how to get particular psychological needs fulfilled in your life in general. For example how you could increase your opportunities to assert yourself, have fun, try new things, or be respected by others.

In order to develop your tools for coping with lowered mood by experimenting with different behavioural responses to daily events in your life, we need to look at another chart that will serve you well along this road. This chart is the Response Record Chart. We have included a blank chart for you to examine and make your own charts, either by copying it also yet to suit your own needs. In addition we have included actual charts from Jane, Susan and Tony that will give you an idea of how they were able to fill in these charts. They successfully experimented with different behavioural responses and set new goals as a result of the feedback that they were able to record on their particular chart.

## TASKS

Your tasks at the end of chapter 8 are:

1. 1.To begin filling in your own response record chart, which will enable you to experiment with different behavioural responses, and confirm that these have had positive results in substantially improving your mood.

2. 2.When people feel unhappy or stressed these emotions tend to lead to thinking biases – we pay extra attention to negative events and overlook positive events.

When we pay extra attention to thinking about what has been going wrong for us, we tend to overestimate how likely it is that our future will be filled with negative events. This in turn leads to us feeling worse. Thinking about "what's gone right" has the opposite effect – we start to expect good things will keep happening to us.

try doing this next time you're in a bad mood, or

try doing this at the end of each day for a week,...

...and see how it affects your thoughts and feelings.

In the long term it might be better to use this technique once a week rather than everyday to avoid becoming bored with it. For example, each Wednesday try writing down three or four things that went right during the past week. An easy way to do this, if you use email a lot, is to write your list in an email and send it to yourself.

It's also a good experiment for couples to do together, (if both people are interested in doing it. Briefly tell your partner three or four things that went right during your day, and they tell you three or four things that went right in their day. Expressing positive emotions to partners tends to make us feel closer to them, even when the things that went right are not relationship related. If you try this experiment with your partner, see whether doing it makes you feel closer to your partner and happier with your life.

If you like it, you might make it a weekly relationship ritual. For example, each Friday night tell each other three or four things that went right in the past week. To reiterate, they do not need to be relationship related, just things that went right in any area of your life.

As before, fill in another mood chart and keep it with the others. By now, you should be able to see a definite upward movement in your recorded moods. If not, don't worry, keep going and it will happen. But if you can see an upwards pattern, that's great. You deserve a pat on the back.

*I usually run three or four times a week now. Pretty boring, but it's so worth it. It's done wonders for my mood.*

*Natalie Portman*

## Response Record Chart

TONY

|  | Situation you wish to test | Normal Response | Desired Outcome | Modified Response | Result |
|---|---|---|---|---|---|
| Sunday | Not go to tanning studio | Go every week | Give it a miss | Go for a walk in the fresh air | Felt a bit shaky |
| Monday | Join a gym | Why? | To get fit? | Try it | Did go, but it was difficult physically |
| Tuesday | Reduce/give up cocaine | Not consider this | To eventually stop | Think seriously about this | Failed |
| Wednesday | Family dinner | Try to get out of | Go, but be more confident | Go, but leave early (business appointment?) | Was a little less stressful |
| Thursday | Lunchtime drink with colleagues | Decline | To go and be sociable | Accept invitation | Was ok |
| Friday | To do and important report—finish without checking | Check it several times | To do it once | Did try | Had to check it once |
| Saturday | Order some healthy food online | Just grab anything | To eat more healthily | Take time to order food | Bought some good food stuff! |

## Response Record Chart                    SUSAN

| | Situation you wish to test | Normal Response | Desired Outcome | Modified Response | Result |
|---|---|---|---|---|---|
| Sunday | To go for a walk | Not interested | To get some exercise | Walk to the shop | Not so bad |
| Monday | Take a small class of Students | Refuse— make an excuse | To get through it | Make sure well prepared | Ok, but not what I like |
| Tuesday | Join the local gym | Probably laugh at the idea | Hope nobody laughs at me | To go, but when the gym is quiet | Did go, but didn't like it much |
| Wednesday | To join a swimming club | Absolutely not | Rather not go, but have to do something | Go for first session as a try out | Ok, but felt very embarrassed |
| Thursday | To go to the hairdresser | A quick trim | To look a bit younger | Asked about a new style | Had some highlights, look quite nice |
| Friday | To listen to another lecturer in the big hall | Not interested | To see how it works | To sit in at the back | The time went quickly— students not too bad |
| Saturday | To go out with friend | Rather stay in | To make the effort | To go for a quiet drink | Actually went out— no panic attack |

## Response Record Chart                    JANE

| | Situation you wish to test | Normal Response | Desired Outcome | Modified Response | Result |
|---|---|---|---|---|---|
| Sunday | Friend asked me to go to dancing | To say no | To go out | Ok, that would be nice | Went out but felt nervous |
| Monday | Husband's check up at doctors | Absolute panic | To go along and keep calm | Try to be positive, he's doing well | Was not as scary as expected |
| Tuesday | Shopping for new clothes | Would not bother | To go and at least look in the shops | Go for just one hour | Didn't buy anything but was quite a nice trip |
| Wednesday | Hair cut | Put off Appointment | To go as booked | It can only look better | It does look better |
| Thursday | Awake in the night | Lie in bed worrying about husband | To stop worrying | Read a good book | Eventually fell asleep |
| Friday | To go shopping on my own | Not do this — worry about husband home alone | To go alone | I'll go, but phone you from the shops | Did go, a bit anxious, but only phoned once |
| Saturday | To try some new make-up | Never do this | At least make an effort | Bought a new lipstick | Felt a bit guilty |

## Response Record Chart

|  | Situation you wish to test | Normal Response | Desired Outcome | Modified Response | Result |
|---|---|---|---|---|---|
| Sunday |  |  |  |  |  |
| Monday |  |  |  |  |  |
| Tuesday |  |  |  |  |  |
| Wednesday |  |  |  |  |  |
| Thursday |  |  |  |  |  |
| Friday |  |  |  |  |  |
| Saturday |  |  |  |  |  |

This part of the book is concerned with the highly important area of self-image. This basic concept is the one that can cause you the most problems in your life. We will record and examine your thoughts on this topic later in the chapter.

# CHAPTER 9: SELF IMAGE

# CHAPTER 9: SELF IMAGE

*Whatever kind of vibe, whatever kind of mood I'm in in the day, if I*
*overthink it then I don't get anything good out of it*

*Dan Donegan*

You need to understand, indeed it is very important that you understand, why your thinking and your self image is the way it is. Firstly, let's look at the negative side of the way we think about ourselves, that of low self-esteem. Why do we have such strong negative beliefs about ourselves? Why do we maintain these beliefs long after it has become clear to us that the beliefs are in no way correct? What we need to undertake is a radical process of re-examining our beliefs. Where necessary challenging the more negative of our beliefs about ourselves and people and things around us, and quite possibly reinforce more positive beliefs about these self same things.

It is highly likely that the core beliefs that we hold we have learned and acquired at a very young age. As we go through life and experience a wide range of events, some of which will undoubtedly be setbacks, we see ourselves as a certain way. If the beliefs that we have acquired along the way tend to be more negative, and the setbacks we suffer are difficult to absorb, it is quite possible that we will see ourselves in a very poor light as stupid, ugly, disliked, and possibly even shunned by our peers. When we reach adulthood it should surely be that the deepening of our knowledge and experience is such that we are able to overturn these fallacious and unhelpful beliefs. However this is often not the case. The tendency is for the person thinking along these lines to take note of those facts and events that appear on the surface to reinforce the negative self belief whilst ignoring other more pertinent facts that would say the opposite. In this way we perpetuate the myth that we have created and learned during childhood.

The way we make sense of the things that happen around us, we call this "information processing", plays a very big part in maintaining low self-esteem. There is so much happening in our environment at any one time, so much information, that to deal with or make sense of all of it is an impossible task. For this reason our brain tends to choose what we pay attention to, and how we think

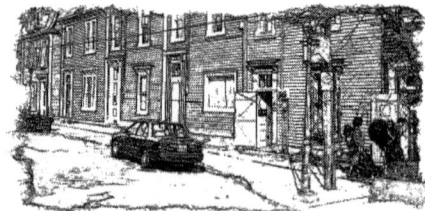

about and make sense of things. Often this is due to the beliefs we hold. We tend to pay attention to things we expect and interpret things in a way that is consistent with our expectations. As a result we tend to remember only things that happen in our lives that are consistent with what we believe to be true. This process of attending to and interpreting things in a manner that is consistent (rather than inconsistent) with our beliefs, is something all human beings do and not just those with problems with low self-esteem.

Let us look at this further using an example not related to self-esteem. You may have the belief your neighbours are noisy. This belief may be based on your experience of the first night they moved into the house next door and had a loud party that kept you awake all hours of the night and early morning. However, your belief about your neighbours, which started from an initial experience, might still remain a few years later because:

- you only pay attention to your neighbours when they are
  noisy, when they are quiet

- you interpret any noise you as coming from those particular
  neighbours, without checking if it is

Whenever the topic of your neighbours comes to mind, you only remember the occasions that they have been noisy. Therefore your original belief "My neighbours are noisy" holds strong.

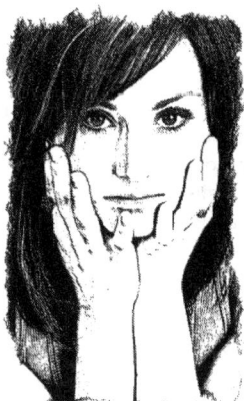

Let us try another example, but this time related to low self-esteem. Let us say your negative core belief is "i am a failure". This is a conclusion you arrive at following certain experiences you had when you were younger. How does this affect your information processing now? Holding the belief you are a failure means that you probably only focus on the times you make mistakes or fail to do something well. You probably ignore any successes, or play them down, "that was a fluke". Also it is unlikely that you acknowledge the times when you have done an acceptable job. Those times are never given a second thought because to you they are "no big deal". Therefore, you only pay attention to negative incidents that confirm your belief that you are a failure. You probably also have quite an extreme view of what success and failure is, with no middle ground. As such, the phrase "I did well" rarely enters your vocabulary. You might easily jump to the extreme conclusion that you have failed at something, when realistically you might not have done too badly at all ("I didn't get an A on the assignment — I'm a complete failure!"). You also tend to interpret the things that happen in your life as confirming your belief that you are a failure when there are likely to be other less harsh interpretations you could make.

The problem is you seem to be always gathering evidence that supports your negative core belief. You only ever pay attention and interpret things in a manner that confirms how you see yourself. In this way, your negative core beliefs are self-fulfilling. 'Once they are in place you will keep gathering information to keep them strong, rarely gathering information to challenge and expose them as biased and inaccurate opinions of yourself.

While the unhelpful rules and assumptions you were introduced to are designed to protect you from the truth of your negative core belief, these also play a part in keeping the core belief alive.

Unhelpful rules and assumptions will tend to affect you behave.

Examples:-

- I must do everything 100% perfectly, or fail

- if you get too close to other people they will reject me

- people won't like me if I express my true feelings and opinions

You will run yourself ragged trying to do everything perfectly, or stay at a comfortable distance from others to avoid rejection. Maybe you will not show anyone the true you in the hope that you will be liked. As long as you do these things, you will probably feel okay about yourself.

The problem is that these rules restrict your behaviour in such a way that you do not have the opportunity to put your negative core beliefs to the test and see if they are true. You never intentionally do a mediocre job and see if dire consequences follow. You never get close to others to see if you really would be rejected. You never express your opinion and see if people still accept you. These rules make us behave in ways that are unhelpful to us. Essentially they stop us from putting ourselves in a position to see if the things we believe about ourselves or to see if the consequences we fear are true. In this way, the rules and assumptions we have limit our opportunities to have experiences that are inconsistent with our negative core beliefs. They restrict us from behaving in ways that allow us to have experiences that would challenge our beliefs and change them. Hence, the unhelpful behaviour that is aimed at meeting our rules and avoiding our assumptions, also keep our negative beliefs about ourselves alive and well. In the previous module, we mentioned that as long as we are able to live up to our rules and assumptions, we might not feel bad about ourselves, but the low self-esteem lies dormant.

Life is full of all sorts of challenges everyday. When these challenges relate to your negative core beliefs and unhelpful rules and assumptions, they become what we would call "at-risk situations" for low self-esteem. These are situations where your rules and assumptions are at risk of being broken or are broken outright. You cannot or will have great difficulty living up to your rules or avoiding your assumptions. Such situations are always going to arise because our rules and assumptions are unrealistic, extreme, and inflexible. Because of the high and often impossible standards that have been set, these rules will always be susceptible to being broken. What happens when we are faced with an at-risk situation? This is when the dormant low self-esteem becomes active. When you encounter an at-risk situation, your negative core belief about yourself is activated, (it goes of like an alarm, lights up like a light bulb, is rekindled like a burning flame). It influences how you think, behave and feel in the situation. When a negative core belief is activated in an at-risk situation, you are likely to think that things will turn out badly or you

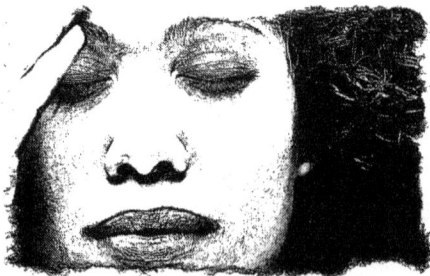

134

become extremely critical of yourself.

We call these two types of thoughts:-

- Biased Expectations
- Negative Self Evaluations

These types of thoughts will then influence how you behave. You might avoid doing certain things.

- try things out but give up when things get too difficult
- take precautions to prevent a negative outcome
- withdraw from situations

This behaviour is unhelpful because it does not address the main issue or solve the problem. Instead leads to negative unhelpful feelings (such as anxiety, frustration, depression, or shame) and confirm the negative core belief. This also causes the negative core belief to remain activated and this time, the low self-esteem is no longer dormant — it is now acute low self-esteem.

Here's an example. Let us say your negative core belief is "I am incompetent" and your unhelpful rule is "I must do everything 100% perfectly, without mistakes, and without the help of others.". As long as you follow your rule,you might feel okay about yourself, because your incompetence is quashed or hidden for the time being. However, Isay you encounter a new and challenging experience — you are starting a new and difficult course of study. You are now in a situation where you are probably unable do things 100% perfectly without mistakes or without the help of others, because the situation you are in is new and challenging, and you lack experience in this area. You are now in an at-risk situation for low self-esteem because your rule is either broken or looks likely to be broken. When this happens, your belief "I am incompetent" is activated, and this belief is brought to the forefront of your mind and now affects how you

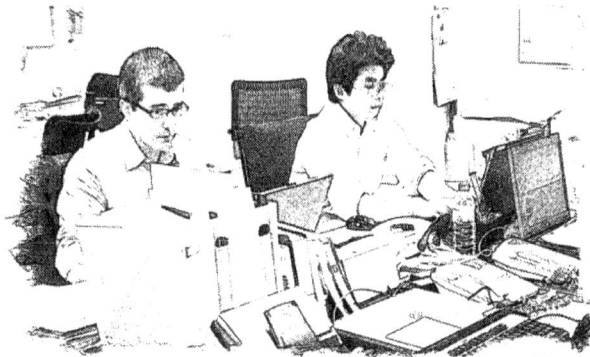

respond in the situation.

If your rule is only threatened (it has not been broken yet, but looks likely to be broken at some point) your response might be to expect things will turn out badly. We call this having biased expectations. This means the way you think is consumed by predicting the worst and jumping to negative conclusions about how the situation will pan out, saying things such as:-

I'm not going to be able to do this.

- I will fail.

- Others will criticise me.

- I won't do a good job.

As a result of having these biased expectations, you might behave in certain ways. You might begin to avoid attending lectures or put assignments off until the last minute. You might become extremely cautious and over-prepared, such as staying up all hours of the night working on an assignment.

Alternatively, you might give the course a try but withdraw when an assignment seems too difficult. We call these three types of behaviours avoidance, taking safety precautions, and escaping. These thoughts and behaviours contribute to you feeling anxious, nervous, tense, afraid, uncertain and doubtful. Your biased expectations, unhelpful behaviours and anxiety may impair your performance confirming to yourself that you were right — "I am incompetent". Your negative core beliefs therefore remain unchanged and continue to be activated. By avoiding things or escaping from difficult situations, you never test out your biased expectations to see if they are accurate. Even if your biased expectations do not come true and things go well, by taking safety precautions you might believe that everything is a close call this time, and that you might not be so lucky next time.

Again, your negative core belief is not changed. So you can see that the way you think and behave in -risk situations leads to unhelpful emotions and maintains your negative beliefs about yourself.

If your rule is actually broken, your response might be to engage in negative self evaluations. This means that the way you think is consumed by self-blame and self-criticism. You become very harsh on yourself, beating yourself up about perceived mistakes or inadequacies saying things such as:-

- I should have done better.

- If I can't even do this, I must be really dumb.

- I knew I didn't have it in me.

- It just shows that.

- I' m really lousy.

Again, as a result you may behave in certain ways:-

- isolating yourself

- withdrawing

- hibernating

- not taking care of yourself

- not doing much

- being passive

- not doing enjoyable things

This is all because you think you don't deserve positive things. When you think and behave in this way you will tend to feel:-

- depressed

- sad

- low

- upset

- dejected

- hopeless

Given that a sign of depression is negative self-talk, these feelings will also tend to keep your negative beliefs about yourself activated.

What then happens is that your negative self-evaluations, unhelpful behavioursand depression all confirm to you that you were right — "I am incompetent". This keeping the belief alive, well after the at-risk situation has passed. So again, you can see that the way you think, behave and feel in at-risk situations, means your negative beliefs gather further support and become even more unwavering.

While it can be helpful to understand how the problems we have today might have developed from our past experiences, it might also be discouraging, because unfortunately we cannot change our past. However, what we have seen in this module is that there are things we do on a day-to-day basis that maintain the negative core beliefs we have about ourselves, keeping them alive and active today.

This is good news, because given that these things happen on a daily basis, you can work on changing them. You can change the negative views you have developed about yourself. This means that things can be different and you can overcome low self-esteem. What is important now is that you commit yourself to making the effort in addressing your unhelpful thinking and unhelpful behaviour from day to day. The rest of the modules in this package will focus on the things that you can start doing to chip away at your low self-esteem. Before long, you will begin to see yourself in a better light and treat yourself more kindly.

The approach taken in this information package of identifying and changing unhelpful thinking and behaviour to overcome low self-esteem comes from a type of treatment known as Cognitive Behavioural Therapy (CBT). This type of psychological treatment has been evaluated scientifically and shown to be effective in treating a number of psychological problems. CBT is aimed at changing your unhelpful thinking patterns and beliefs (the cognitive part), as well as any unhelpful style of behaving (the behavioural part). This will bring about a change in how you see yourself and how you feel.

## CORE BELIEF CHALLENGE CHART

(Choose a belief that you feel is worth examining. This could be in relation to your work, yourself, your friends and acquaintances and friends, your diet, your fitness plan etc. In fact anything that YOU feel is important to you. E.g. "although I am fairly overweight, I do not believe that it is worth going through the hassle of losing weight" or "I believe that the people at work are overly critical of the work I do." Then write down WHY you believe this to be true. Then write down reasonable alternatives to your beliefs. Finally, write down which of these beliefs is substantially justified, and why.)

1.

    a.    Core Belief

    b.    Why I hold this belief to be true

    c.    Reasonable alternative beliefs

    d.    Which belief is more realistic, and why

2.

    a.    Core Belief

    b.    Why I hold this belie¬f to be true

    c.    Reasonable alternative beliefs

    d.    Which belief is more realistic, and why

3.

    a.    Core Belief

    b.    Why I hold this belief to be true

    c.    Reasonable alternative beliefs

    d.    Which belief is more realistic, and why

4.

    a.    Core Belief

    b.    Why I hold this belief to be true

    c.    Reasonable alternative beliefs

    d.    Which belief is more realistic, and why

# SELF IMAGE

Core Belief Summary Chart                    week ending .........................................

| Core Beliefs I Am Working On This Week | Re-evaluated this belief? YES/NO |
|---|---|
|  |  |
|  |  |
|  |  |
|  |  |
|  |  |
|  |  |
|  |  |
|  |  |
|  |  |

There are things that we do everyday that maintain our negative core beliefs, long after the negative experiences that generated them have passed.

Low self-esteem is maintained by:-

- The way we process information in our environment (our attention and interpretation).

- What our unhelpful rules and assumptions generate (no opportunity to put negative core beliefs to the test).

- Our responses in 'At-Risk Situations' (biased expectations and negative self-evaluations).

- 'At-Risk Situations' are situations where your unhelpful rules and assumptions are at risk of being broken or are broken outright. When this occurs, negative core beliefs and dormant low self-esteem become activated.

- When your negative core beliefs are activated, they lead you to either expect that things will not turn out well (biased expectations) or become highly critical of yourself (negative self-evaluations). Both types of thoughts will lead you to engage in unhelpful behaviours and feel unhelpful emotions such as anxiety or depression

- The unhelpful thoughts, behaviours and feelings that are generated from 'At-Risk Situations' confirm your negative view of yourself and keep it alive. Therefore, these responses maintain your negative beliefs about yourself over the long-term.

Overcoming low self-esteem involves addressing the factors in the here-and-now that maintain low self-esteem. The strategies used to address these factors come from a style of therapy known as Cognitive Behavioural Therapy (CBT), which involves changing unhelpful thinking and behaviour patterns to change how you feel.

In this chapter we have introduced two further charts, the core belief challenge chart and the core beliefs summary chart. Then, using if necessary information that you have recorded previously in your thought record and mood record charts, begin filling in your own charts so that you can begin to see how the system works.

Your belief system gives you a framework that helps you interpret and understand the experiences you face in life. A belief is something you accept as true, without question. That means you can expect that every day it will seem just as true as it was the day before. Your beliefs are deeply embedded in you, so you, and particularly your team of protective inner selves, live your life around them, without thinking, questioning or even being aware of them.

The beliefs that helped you survive and fit into your childhood will have been unique for you and different from mine (unless the toughest things you and I had to cope with were very similar). If in childhood I was told I would always fail, a core belief might be "I can't". This helps me because it gives me a framework around which to survive, a map of the world that helps me cope with life and plan my future. Now I know what to expect in life and I can start learning how best to fit into my unbalanced family system.

So our core beliefs, as they took root in our first few years, became a kind of

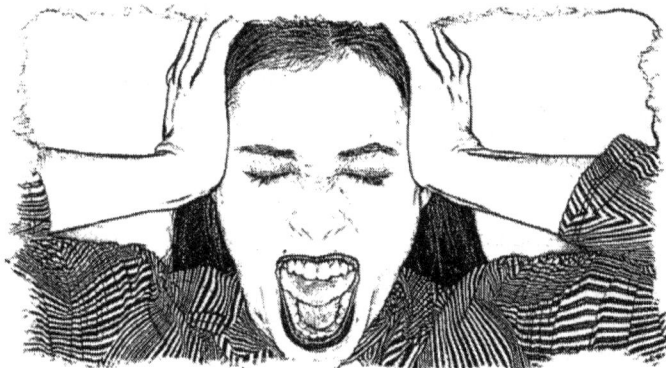

summary of the most basic convictions we make up about our self-worth. The kind of person we are, what will become of us as a result, our place in the family and the world and how we can expect others to treat us all through our lifetime.

Core beliefs like these are supported by the primary inner self system. This means they grow stronger rather than weaker. One of the ways they often grow is by helping make sense of our worst childhood experiences, in the only way a small child can, by telling us that what went wrong was essentially our fault. Even though this assumption was based on false information, or false understandings set up in early childhood, it becomes more firmly established as you grow up. Today it may still shape and guide much of our life and the way we react to those around us. It also provides us with an unusual gift in the way it motivates us to change our natural personality and adapt to become more like the person others want us to be.

These beliefs about yourself, which you hold onto so strongly also reflect your deepest vulnerability and pain and help to keep these locked within you.

## CORE BELIEFS RESONATE THROUGH YOUR WHOLE LIFE

Your strongest inner and polarised selves were created to help you live with your core beliefs. Unfortunately while they were helping you live with a negative core belief these same selves, in conjunction with your supporting beliefs, were also making it seem as if that belief really must have been true.

Your locked in automatic repetitive behaviour patterns set up by your polarised selves certainly helped you cope with the pain of your unbalanced beliefs, but they also created a binding situation. Learning to live with, and constantly find better ways to cope with these false beliefs, gave you no opportunity to discover ways to question or to change them.

Instead, what you and I have learned for most of our life, so far, is simply how to channel all our energy and resources towards dealing with these negative beliefs.

"Money, time, relationships, professional skills, family, everything has been reorganised so that it can be better used to distance me from my pain, my vulnerability and my fear of my negative beliefs getting any worse than they already are. In so doing I also distance myself from the love that I am so desperately seeking". (Nikki Nemerouf)

Your senses are so tied up, bound and distorted by the false belief that you literally cannot see the positive reality in front of you. You may even fight it when someone else tries to show you that these beliefs have a positive side, until you begin the process called balancing and transformation, as explained at the end of this section.

Whatever your unbalanced beliefs are, they help to define your unique and individual core issues and these in turn control the way your inner selves react when those issues are triggered. It has often been said that whatever your most negative core belief about yourself might be, that is the one your selves will tend most to "dance around". There are hundreds of core issues and core beliefs, so you can expect that yours may be quite different from those held by the person next to you.

Examples of negative core beliefs or feelings about myself:-

- not good enough (incompetent)
- not good enough (unlovable)
- unwanted, different
- defective, imperfect, bad
- powerless, one-below
- in danger, not safe
- don't know, wrong

Examples of life Issue related to core belief:-

- success
- love
- belonging
- self worth
- control
- security

# NEGATIVE CORE BELIEFS

I am no good

I can't get it right

I can't make it work (klutz)

I can't fix it

I am not good enough

I am unsuccessful

I'm not valuable

I am inferior

I am nothing

I am worthless

I am invisible

I am insignificant

Not good enough (unlovable)

I am not lovable

I am unacceptable

I am plain and dull

I am not special

I don't matter

I am unworthy

I am not interesting enough

Don't know, wrong

I don't know

I get it wrong

I am always wrong

I can't understand

I'm not understood

I am in the wrong place

I am no good

I am a mistake

In danger or not safe

I'm not safe

I am afraid

I am uncertain

I am vulnerable

I am helpless

Unwanted, different

I don't belong

I am unwanted

I am alone

I am unwelcome

I don't fit in anywhere

I don't exist

I'm nothing

I should not be here at all

I'm not anybody

I am left out

I am unsuitable

I am uninteresting

I am unimportant

I don't matter

Defective, imperfect, bad

It's my fault

I am guilty

I am bad

I am not whole

I am imperfect

I am unattractive

I am flawed

I am stupid

I am awkward

I am slow

I can't be me

I'm not true

I'm dirty

I am ugly

I am fat

I'm shameful

I am unclean

I am useless

I am crazy

I have a mental problem

I am out of control

I can't make myself clear

I am mistaken

I am unbalanced

I will fail

I am a failure

I don't deserve to be loved

I don't deserve to be cared for

I don't deserve anything

There's something wrong with me

Powerless, one-below

I can't do it

I can't

I am a victim

I am weak

I am powerless

I am a failure

I am ineffective

I don't have any choice

I am less than

I am helpless

I finish last

I am always number two

I am always one-below

I can't stand up for myself

I am inferior

I am a loser

I am inadequate

I can't say 'no'

Now, take one or more core belief challenge charts, as you feel are required, and fill them in with each of the negative beliefs that you have ticked. Then go through the process of working through each negative belief, changing it and writing down a more realistic assessment of your own situation. Do this exercise as often as you require. We need hardly add that without question the personal view you hold of yourself is wrong in many respects. Only by challenging your beliefs will you come to realise both how incorrect is your thinking about yourself, but also what is a more truthful way of thinking about the very qualities that you do possess.

You should also bear in mind that while you are challenging and correcting some of your false negative beliefs, you need to take steps to ensure that you equip yourself to avoid making the kinds of false assumptions that lead in this negative direction. Here are a few simple rules of thumb for you to apply as you go through each and every day. It would be very helpful for you to write them on a separate sheet of paper or piece of card and keep it handy for you to refer to now and again. There are six rules in all. If while you are evaluating your core beliefs you find that there is a common thread to the false assumptions that you have made, write this down as well as a reminder to yourself not to continue falling into the same trap.

- Remember that the only safe assumption to make is that your first assumptions might be false. This keeps your head level and your mind open.

- Recognise the assumptions you make in everyday life and think about whether they are useful. Throw out anything that does not help you live and work more efficiently.

- Respect other people's ideas. Even though you might disagree with someone else on a hot topic, recognise that their opinion is not worthless simply because it's not the same as your own.

- Be as objective as you can in making evaluative decisions. Whether you're at work, at home or with your friends, be as logical and fair as possible in your judgments.

- Resist the urge to accept stereotypes. Even though they might be accurate, stereotypes can cloud your judgment.

- Base your judgments only on the most apparent facts. This is the most logical way of doing things and it will stop you from make false assumptions altogether.

If you look deep inside yourself you will find that some of the beliefs no longer support you in your cause or should I say greater goal. Just looking at your potential and thinking "I wonder what can I achieve if I change a few of my core beliefs". Life would start appearing more meaningful. It's all about you believing in whatever you want to believe. Trust me the results will more than surprise you, of course in a positive way.

Here is a wonderful story that we hope will inspire you to think along the right lines.

# SELF IMAGE

Two men, both seriously ill, occupied the same hospital room. One man was allowed to sit up in his bed for an hour a day to drain the fluids from his lungs. His bed was next to the room's only window. The other man had to spend all his time flat on his back.

The men talked for hours on end. They spoke of their wives and families, homes, jobs, involvement in the military service and where they had been on vacation. Every afternoon when the man in the bed next to the window could sit up, he would pass the time by describing to his roommate all the things he could see outside the window.

The man in the other bed would live for those one hour periods where his world would be broadened and enlivened by all the activity and colour of the outside world. The window overlooked a park with a lovely lake, the man had said. Ducks and swans played on the water while children sailed their model boats. Lovers walked arm in arm amid flowers of every colour of the rainbow. Grand old trees graced the landscape and a fine view of the city skyline could be seen in the distance. As the man by the window described all this in exquisite detail, the man on the other side of the room would close his eyes and imagine the picturesque scene.

One warm afternoon the man by the window described a parade passing by. Although the other man could not hear the band, he could see it in his mind's eye as the gentleman by the window portrayed it with descriptive words. Unexpectedly, an alien thought entered his head "Why should he have all the pleasure of seeing everything while I never get to see anything?". It didn't seem fair. As the thought fermented, the man felt ashamed at first. But as the days passed and he missed seeing more sights, his envy eroded into resentment and soon turned him sour. He began to brood and found himself unable to sleep. He should be by that window, and that thought now controlled his life.

Late one night, as he lay staring at the ceiling, the man by the window began to cough. He was choking on the fluid in his lungs. The other man watched in the dimly lit room as the struggling man by the window groped for the button to call for help. Listening from across the room, he never moved, never pushed his own button which would have brought the nurse running. In less than five minutes, the coughing and choking stopped, along with the sound of breathing. Now, there was only silence–deathly silence.

The following morning, the day nurse arrived to bring water for their baths. When she found the lifeless body of the man by the window, she was saddened and called the hospital attendant to take it away–no words, no fuss. As soon as it seemed appropriate, the man asked if he could be moved next to the window. The nurse was happy to make the switch and after making sure he was comfortable, she left him alone.

Slowly, painfully, he propped himself up on one elbow to take his first look. Finally, he would have the joy of seeing it all himself. He strained to slowly turn to look out the window beside the bed.

It faced a blank wall.

Whether it is for yourself or to benefit other people, which surely also benefit you, you need to keep working at challenging and where necessary modifying your core beliefs. Someone with what is often called a "can do" attitude finds a way to tackle any problem, resolve any issue. That person is energetic, determined and motivated. Projects are begun and finished. The "can do" person is the "go to" person.

The "I can..." person finds solutions and possibilities. What others consider failures, the "I can" person considers learning opportunities, opportunities for problem solving, adventures.

The "I can't" person sees only roadblocks.

Task for the end of chapter 9: We have introduced you to two new charts. You may use your mood and thought charts as a guide to fill in as many of the new Core Belief Challenge Charts as you are able. Then, take a Core Belief Summary Chart, just one, and fill it in ONLY with the most important (to you) Core Beliefs that you need to re-evaluate. Use this Summary Chart as a guide for the future.

## TASKS

By now, you are used to the process of filling in the Mood Compass. You know what to do!

*Although there is a great deal of controversy among scientists about the effects of ingested food on the brain, no one denies that you can change your cognition and mood by what you eat.*

*Arthur Winter*

This chapter deals with the tough problem of depression. You will learn how to identify key problems and learn to develop strategies to deal with them. The symptoms are many and it is often easy to discount depression as one of many other problems.

# CHAPTER 10: DEPRESSION

# CHAPTER 10: DEPRESSION

*Saying that positive thinking usually doesn't work is such heresy that I may be unceremoniously drummed out of the personal development field. And, it is mostly true.*

*Robert White*

In everyone's lives they will inevitably encounter a degree of sadness. This could occur very few times or in some people much more frequently. Society has chosen to label deep sadness as an acknowledged illness caused Depression. This illness can stay with the sufferer for a very lengthy period. It was even recognised in ancient times by the Greeks, who acknowledged how serious this illness could be. They also noted that in certain individuals the natural lifting of sadness was less likely to occur and they tended to remain sad or dejected.

If you have yourself suffered from the dark depths of black despair of depression, or possibly even had a close relation or acquaintance who has suffered in this way, you will be aware of how serious this illness can be and how difficult it can be to cure. In Victorian times depression in women was known as an attack of the Vapours. In the early 20th century a man would be directed to "act like a man" or a woman told to "shake yourself out of it". Depression is an illness about which little has been known until more recently.

The reality is that depression is nothing whatever to do with "acting like a man" or "shake yourself out of it". Indeed it has more to do with brain chemistry. Recent suggestions are that changes in nerve pathways and brain chemicals called neurotransmitters can affect moods and thoughts to the point where they can in certain individuals cause depression.

Symptoms of depression can include:-

- insomnia
- decreased appetite
- increased appetite
- extreme agitation or lethargy
- generally a feeling of apathy

There has also been additional scientific evidence to suggest that a combination of genetic factors can be more prevalent in those prone to bouts of depression.

Brain chemistry and neurotransmitters however are not the complete reason for the onset of depression. The reasons are undoubtedly many and varied. It would by no means be unreasonable to suggest a combination of nature and nurture life behind most incidences of depression.

# DEPRESSION

Then again there are events in people's lives that frequently bring on depression:-

- bereavement
- redundancy
- severe illness either in oneself or in a loved one
- the time of year (SAD)

This illness known as SAD (Seasonal Affective Disorder) is where sufferers tend to experience depression in the darker winter months. Scientists have speculated that this is due to a lack of sunlight, although this is yet to be proven.

Often there is not one factor or event that causes a person to suffer depression. Any combination of or indeed just one single one can be responsible. According to the National Institute of Mental Health, the number of adults who suffer from depression could be as many as one in ten. There is also an increasing incidence of depression in young people. This is possibly caused by environmental factors, such as the isolation of the computer age, making those more prone to the illness of depression likely to experience the actual illness.

What is unarguable is that the experience of depression takes a very heavy toll of the person concerned, and often those around them. It is an illness that needs to be taken seriously and all efforts made to assist the sufferer to find a means of relieving the symptoms. At this stage we would suggest that you fill in the following questionnaire which will give you a good indication as to the likelihood or otherwise of your suffering from depression. The maximum possible score is 90, which would be a very severely depressed individual indeed. If your score is 45 or more it is possible that you are suffering from depression. However, the most value you will get out of this depression questionnaire is to fill it in on a weekly basis. Then you can compare your mood from week to week and see if it is in fact improving or worsening and then act accordingly.

Goldberg Depression Questionnaire. Use this questionnaire to help determine if you are likely to be suffering from depression, or to monitor your mood.

Instructions: You might reproduce this scale and use it on a weekly basis to track your moods. It also might be used to show your doctor how your symptoms have changed from one visit to the next. Changes of five or more points are significant. This scale is not designed to make a diagnosis of depression or take the place of a professional diagnosis. If you suspect that you are depressed, please consult with a mental health professional as soon as possible.

## Goldberg Depression Questionnaire

Read through each question and tick on the option that best described you. Refer to the last page for scoring and analysis information.

**1. I do things slowly.**

Not at all ☐

Just a little ☐

Somewhat ☐

Moderately ☐

Quite a lot ☐

Very much ☐

**2. My future seems hopeless**

Not at all ☐

Just a little ☐

Somewhat ☐

Moderately ☐

Quite a lot ☐

Very much ☐

# DEPRESSION

### 3. It is hard for me to concentrate on reading.

Not at all ☐

Just a little ☐

Somewhat ☐

Moderately ☐

Quite a lot ☐

Very much ☐

### 4. The pleasure and joy has gone out of my life.

Not at all ☐

Just a little ☐

Somewhat ☐

Moderately ☐

Quite a lot ☐

Very much ☐

### 5. I have difficulty making decision s.

Not at all ☐

Just a little ☐

Somewhat ☐

Moderately ☐

Quite a lot ☐

Very much ☐

**6. I have lost interest in aspects of life that used to be important to me.**

First Answer ☐

Second Answer ☐

Third Answer ☐

Fourth Answer ☐

Fifth Answer ☐

Sixth Answer ☐

**7. I feel sad, blue and unhappy.**

Not at all ☐

Just a little ☐

Somewhat ☐

Moderately ☐

Quite a lot ☐

Very much ☐

**8. I am agitated and keep moving around.**

Not at all ☐

Just a little ☐

Somewhat ☐

Moderately ☐

Quite a lot ☐

Very much ☐

# DEPRESSION

**9. I feel fatigued.**

First Answer ☐

Second Answer ☐

Third Answer ☐

Fourth Answer ☐

Fifth Answer ☐

Sixth Answer ☐

**10. It takes great effort for me to do simple things.**

Not at all ☐

Just a little ☐

Somewhat ☐

Moderately ☐

Quite a lot ☐

Very much ☐

**11. I feel I am a guilty person who deserves to be punished.**

Not at all ☐

Just a little ☐

Somewhat ☐

Moderately ☐

Quite a lot ☐

Very much ☐

**12. I feel like a failure.**

First Answer ☐

Second Answer ☐

Third Answer ☐

Fourth Answer ☐

Fifth Answer ☐

Sixth Answer ☐

**13. I feel lifeless — more dead than alive.**

Not at all ☐

Just a little ☐

Somewhat ☐

Moderately ☐

Quite a lot ☐

Very much ☐

**14. My sleep has been disturbed—too little, too much or broken sleep.**

Not at all ☐

Just a little ☐

Somewhat ☐

Moderately ☐

Quite a lot ☐

Very much ☐

# DEPRESSION

### 15. I spent time thinking about HOW I might kill myself.

First Answer ☐

Second Answer ☐

Third Answer ☐

Fourth Answer ☐

Fifth Answer ☐

Sixth Answer ☐

### 16. I feel trapped or caught.

Not at all ☐

Just a little ☐

Somewhat ☐

Moderately ☐

Quite a lot ☐

Very much ☐

### 17. I feel depressed even when good things happen to me.

Not at all ☐

Just a little ☐

Somewhat ☐

Moderately ☐

Quite a lot ☐

Very much ☐

**18. Without trying to diet, I have lost, or gained, weight.**

First Answer

Second Answer

Third Answer

Fourth Answer

Fifth Answer

Sixth Answer

Add up all your points to obtain a total score

- Not at all = 0
- Just a little = 1 point
- Somewhat = 2 points
- Moderately = 3 points
- Quite a lot = 4 points
- Very much = 5 points

Find your total score on the Interpretation Table below

Score Interpretation

| | |
|---|---|
| 54 and up | Severely Clinically Depressed |
| 36 - 53 | Clinically Depressed, Moderate - Severe |
| 22 - 35 | Clinically Depressed, Mild - Moderate |
| 18 - 21 | Borderline Clinical Depression |
| 10 - 17 | Possibly Mildly Depressed |
| 0 - 9 | No Depression Likely |

# DEPRESSION

Think back to Jane who we introduced in Chapter 1, a patient that we were able to help find the symptoms that she suffered after the mild heart attack of her husband. Jane reported to us that she felt constantly tired. She had given up her leisure activities to concentrate on looking after her husband, who she wrongly perceived as being at risk of premature death. In this respect she was able to identify that, in some perverse way, she felt that she was guilty of failing to adequately look after her husband and needed to be punished. She had gained weight, failed to look after her appearance and generally lost interest in most of those aspects of her life that used to be important to her, primarily her dancing classes. It is clear that were she to take the depression questionnaire when she first came to see us, she would have scored relatively highly, quite possibly even extremely highly. Whilst the questionnaire itself should not be used as an absolute final assessment of depression, it should be used as an aid to diagnosis as an indicator. This is especially true for the person that fills in these questionnaires on a regular basis to assess the progress of their illness.

Bipolar Disorder, which used to be called Manic Depression, involves both periods of feeling low (depressed) and high (mania). Most people experience a range of moods depending on what is happening in their lives. When good things happen, such as starting a new job, going on a holiday or falling in love, it's natural to feel happy. On the other hand, when there are difficulties, losing a job or a loved one, having money or family problems, it can make a person feel down. However, people with bipolar disorder experience extreme moods that can change regularly. These may not relate to what is happening in their lives, although their mood swings may be triggered by certain events.

A person with bipolar disorder will have symptoms of both depression and mania at different times. The lists of symptoms below will not provide a diagnosis - only a doctor can do that. They will however, help you understand if you, or someone close to you, may have symptoms of bipolar disorder. If you notice any behavioural changes that last for more than two weeks in close family or friends, then it is worth asking if the person may be depressed. Keeping mood records and charts will greatly help in this kind of assessment.

Common behaviour associated with depression includes:-

- moodiness that is out of character

- increased irritability and frustration

- finding it hard to take minor personal criticisms

- spending less time with friends and family

- loss of interest in food, sex, exercise or other pleasurable activities

- being awake throughout the night

- increased alcohol and drug use

- staying home from work or school

- increased physical health complaints like fatigue or pain

- being reckless or taking unnecessary risks (e.g. driving fast or dangerously)
- slowing down of thoughts and actions

Common behaviour associated with mania includes:-

- increased energy
- irritability
- overactivity
- increased spending
- increased sex drive
- racing thoughts
- rapid speech
- decreased sleep
- grandiose ideas
- hallucinations and/or delusions

Some people with bipolar disorder also have symptoms of psychosis. These include:-

- hallucinations - (seeing or hearing things or people that are not there)
- paranoia - (feeling everyone is against them)
- delusions – (having beliefs that are not based on reality)

Bipolar disorder can be influenced by a range of factors. It seems to be most closely linked to family history. For example, while bipolar disorder affects around 2 per cent of the general population at some stage of their lives, people who have a parent with bipolar disorder have a 10 per cent chance of having the illness themselves.

## ENVIRONMENTAL FACTORS

While a major cause of bipolar disorder seems to be genetic, stress can also trigger symptoms. Common triggers include:-

- changing jobs
- changing living arrangements
- family and relationship problems
- being the victim of verbal, sexual, physical or emotional abuse or trauma
- other life transitions e.g. having a child
- death or loss of someone close

# DEPRESSION

Physical health issues which can also trigger bipolar disorder include:-

- pregnancy and childbirth
- hormonal problems (hyper and hypothyroidism)
- brain problems (Parkinson's and Huntington's disease)
- autoimmune problems (Lupus, HIV)
- cancer

Most people feel bad about themselves from time to time. Temporary feelings of low self-esteem may be triggered by being treated poorly by someone else recently or in the past, or by a person's own judgments of him or herself. Low self-esteem is a constant companion for too many people, especially those who experience depression. If you go through life feeling bad about yourself needlessly, low self-esteem keeps you from enjoying life, doing the things you want to do and working toward personal goals.

Let's look back at Susan, who came to us suffering from very low self-esteem which manifested itself in panic attacks and generalised anxiety when she was faced with the prospect of teaching a class of students. As a result of this she was undoubtedly suffering from a substantial degree of depression which we were able to help her treat. Looking at the results for her depression questionnaire the degree of her depression was unmistakable.

## Goldberg Depression Questionnaire

Read through each question and tick on the option that best described you. Refer to the last page for scoring and analysis information.

# SUSAN

**1. I do things slowly.**

Not at all ☐

Just a little ☐

Somewhat ☐

Moderately ☐

Quite a lot ☒

Very much ☐

**2. My future seems hopeless**

Not at all ☐

Just a little ☐

Somewhat ☐

Moderately ☒

Quite a lot ☐

Very much ☐

# DEPRESSION

### 3. It is hard for me to concentrate on reading.

Not at all ☐

Just a little ☐

Somewhat ☒

Moderately ☐

Quite a lot ☐

Very much ☐

### 4. The pleasure and joy has gone out of my life.

Not at all ☐

Just a little ☐

Somewhat ☐

Moderately ☐

Quite a lot ☐

Very much ☒

### 5. I have difficulty making decision s.

Not at all ☐

Just a little ☐

Somewhat ☐

Moderately ☐

Quite a lot ☒

Very much ☐

**6. I have lost interest in aspects of life that used to be important to me.**

First Answer ☐

Second Answer ☐

Third Answer ☐

Fourth Answer ☐

Fifth Answer ☒

Sixth Answer ☐

**7. I feel sad, blue and unhappy.**

Not at all ☐

Just a little ☐

Somewhat ☐

Moderately ☐

Quite a lot ☐

Very much ☒

**8. I am agitated and keep moving around.**

Not at all ☐

Just a little ☐

Somewhat ☐

Moderately ☒

Quite a lot ☐

Very much ☐

# DEPRESSION

### 9. I feel fatigued.

First Answer ☐

Second Answer ☐

Third Answer ☐

Fourth Answer ☒

Fifth Answer ☐

Sixth Answer ☐

### 10. It takes great effort for me to do simple things.

Not at all ☐

Just a little ☐

Somewhat ☐

Moderately ☐

Quite a lot ☐

Very much ☒

### 11. I feel I am a guilty person who deserves to be punished.

Not at all ☐

Just a little ☐

Somewhat ☐

Moderately ☐

Quite a lot ☒

Very much ☐

**12. I feel like a failure.**

First Answer ☐

Second Answer ☐

Third Answer ☐

Fourth Answer ☒

Fifth Answer ☐

Sixth Answer ☐

**13. I feel lifeless — more dead than alive.**

Not at all ☐

Just a little ☐

Somewhat ☐

Moderately ☐

Quite a lot ☐

Very much ☒

**14. My sleep has been disturbed—too little, too much or broken sleep.**

Not at all ☐

Just a little ☐

Somewhat ☐

Moderately ☐

Quite a lot ☒

Very much ☐

# DEPRESSION

**15. I spent time thinking about HOW I might kill myself.**

First Answer ☐

Second Answer ☐

Third Answer ☐

Fourth Answer ☒

Fifth Answer ☐

Sixth Answer ☐

**16. I feel trapped or caught.**

Not at all ☐

Just a little ☐

Somewhat ☐

Moderately ☒

Quite a lot ☐

Very much ☐

**17. I feel depressed even when good things happen to me.**

Not at all ☐

Just a little ☐

Somewhat ☒

Moderately ☐

Quite a lot ☐

Very much ☐

**18. Without trying to diet, I have lost, or gained, weight.**

First Answer ☐

Second Answer ☐

Third Answer ☐

Fourth Answer ☐

Fifth Answer ☐

Sixth Answer ☒

Add up all your points to obtain a total score

- Not at all       =       0
- Just a little    =       1       point
- Somewhat         =       2       points
- Moderately       =       3       points
- Quite a lot      =       4       points
- Very much        =       5       points

Find your total score on the Interpretation Table below

Score Interpretation

54 and up       Severely Clinically Depressed

36 - 53         Clinically Depressed, Moderate - Severe

22 - 35         Clinically Depressed, Mild - Moderate

18 - 21         Borderline Clinical Depression

10 - 17         Possibly Mildly Depressed

0 - 9   No Depression Likely

SCORE         **67**

# DEPRESSION

[[INSERT 1 DEPRESSION QUESTIONNAIRE (COMPLETED FOR SUSAN - MAKE IT LOOK BAD)]]

There are a number of ways that you can immediately employ to remedy low self-esteem.

For example, you could make a simple list of your strengths which will serve as a reminder to yourself that you are a person who possesses considerable strengths. Here is one such possible list:-

- At least five of your strengths, persistence, courage, friendliness, creativity etc.

- At least five things you admire about yourself, for example, the way you have raised your children, your good relationship with someone in your family or your spirituality.

- The five greatest achievements in your life so far, maybe recovering from a serious illness, graduating from high school or learning to use a computer.

- At least twenty other accomplishments — they can be as simple as learning to tie your shoes or to getting an advanced college degree.

- Ten ways to treat or reward yourself that do not include food and that costs nothing, such as walking In woods, window-shopping or chatting with a friend.

- Ten things you can do to make yourself laugh.

- Ten things you could do to help someone else.

- Things that you do that make you feel good about yourself.

Another tip is to accept that we each control our lives. We create our future by effort. No one can do it for us. Unfortunately, most people are looking for instant this, instant that, instant success and instant cash. Well, in our world today the only thing you can get instantly is failure. No one wants to work for their success! So what do they do? They give up! Why? Because it is so much easier to fail than to succeed! Take back the control of your life you deserve success as much as the next person. You just have to accept that you deserve it.

In Susan's particular case she did use a list of this kind to help her realise that further low self-esteem and very negative feelings about herself were in fact quite wrong. When she was able to come to this conclusion, she then found herself able to effectively make use of the charting tools that we have described in earlier chapters to keep a regular weekly record of her progress. In this way she could monitor her moods and thoughts and correct the thinking and assumptions that were central to her low self-esteem, as well as the deep depression that she suffered as a result. Lifting core beliefs and assumptions about yourself can be very difficult, but when you see unmistakable evidence of the progress that you have made and continue to make, the conclusion is unmistakable.

In the case of Tony, the successful business professional, the reasons for his problems were made much more complex with his use of cocaine. Initially he had begun to use cocaine at a stage when he felt the demands of his job were more than he could easily and comfortably cope with. So he used the drug as a boost to keep him on top of things. He came to us with the classic symptoms of depression. He was losing weight and had lost much of his appetite. His morale and personal well-being were constantly undermined by his feelings that his colleagues were looking at him in a very derogatory way. He suffered from insomnia and even when he was able to sleep found that this sleep was interrupted by nightmares. His symptoms were of undoubted depression and when we discuss this with him, together with his difficulties at work and drug habit, his question was what was the main cause of the problem. Was cocaine the cause of the problem? Was his drug habit causing him feelings of paranoia and insomnia? Or was it the problems of paranoia and insomnia that had caused him to begin taking drugs in the first place to enhance his business performance?

During discussions with Tony we were able to help him to come to terms with his problems and to realise that they were rather more complex than a simple yes or no answer as to which of his difficulties came first. We said at the start of this chapter, the reasons for depression very complex and a result of a number of factors. However, in effect the question of what came first was not really very relevant. Any reasonably well informed person knows that the long-term effects of a drug habit can only be ruinous. In terms of his difficulties at work it was not quite so clear. However, once Tony was able to look at his mood charts, thought charts and other records of his feelings he was able to understand more clearly the deep rooted nature of the problem. He did in fact fill in a questionnaire and it became clear that the indications from this questionnaire were that it was quite likely he was suffering from depression. Furthermore it may well have been the case that the depression was the reason for his problems rather than the cocaine which was an attempt to alleviate them or the paranoia and insomnia which were the effects of his low mood.

## Goldberg Depression Questionnaire

Read through each question and tick on the option that best described you.  Refer to the last page for scoring and analysis information.

# TONY

**1.  I do things slowly.**

Not at all ☐

Just a little ☐

Somewhat ☒

Moderately ☐

Quite a lot ☐

Very much ☐

**2.  My future seems hopeless**

Not at all ☐

Just a little ☒

Somewhat ☐

Moderately ☐

Quite a lot ☐

Very much ☐

**3. It is hard for me to concentrate on reading.**

Not at all [X]

Just a little [ ]

Somewhat [ ]

Moderately [ ]

Quite a lot [ ]

Very much [ ]

**4. The pleasure and joy has gone out of my life.**

Not at all [ ]

Just a little [ ]

Somewhat [ ]

Moderately [X]

Quite a lot [ ]

Very much [ ]

**5. I have difficulty making decision s.**

Not at all [ ]

Just a little [ ]

Somewhat [ ]

Moderately [X]

Quite a lot [ ]

Very much [ ]

# DEPRESSION

**6. I have lost interest in aspects of life that used to be important to me.**

First Answer ☐

Second Answer ☐

Third Answer ☐

Fourth Answer ☐

Fifth Answer ☐

Sixth Answer ☒

**7. I feel sad, blue and unhappy.**

Not at all ☐

Just a little ☐

Somewhat ☒

Moderately ☐

Quite a lot ☐

Very much ☐

**8. I am agitated and keep moving around.**

Not at all ☐

Just a little ☐

Somewhat ☐

Moderately ☒

Quite a lot ☐

Very much ☐

**9. I feel fatigued.**

First Answer ☐

Second Answer ☒

Third Answer ☐

Fourth Answer ☐

Fifth Answer ☐

Sixth Answer ☐

**10. It takes great effort for me to do simple things.**

Not at all ☐

Just a little ☐

Somewhat ☐

Moderately ☒

Quite a lot ☐

Very much ☐

**11. I feel I am a guilty person who deserves to be punished.**

Not at all ☐

Just a little ☐

Somewhat ☐

Moderately ☒

Quite a lot ☐

Very much ☐

# DEPRESSION

**12. I feel like a failure.**

First Answer ☐

Second Answer ☐

Third Answer ☒

Fourth Answer ☐

Fifth Answer ☐

Sixth Answer ☐

**13. I feel lifeless — more dead than alive.**

Not at all ☐

Just a little ☐

Somewhat ☒

Moderately ☐

Quite a lot ☐

Very much ☐

**14. My sleep has been disturbed—too little, too much or broken sleep.**

Not at all ☐

Just a little ☐

Somewhat ☒

Moderately ☐

Quite a lot ☐

Very much ☐

**15. I spent time thinking about HOW I might kill myself.**

| | |
|---|---|
| First Answer | ☐ |
| Second Answer | ☒ |
| Third Answer | ☐ |
| Fourth Answer | ☐ |
| Fifth Answer | ☐ |
| Sixth Answer | ☐ |

**16. I feel trapped or caught.**

| | |
|---|---|
| Not at all | ☐ |
| Just a little | ☒ |
| Somewhat | ☐ |
| Moderately | ☐ |
| Quite a lot | ☐ |
| Very much | ☐ |

**17. I feel depressed even when good things happen to me.**

| | |
|---|---|
| Not at all | ☐ |
| Just a little | ☐ |
| Somewhat | ☐ |
| Moderately | ☐ |
| Quite a lot | ☒ |
| Very much | ☐ |

# DEPRESSION

**18. Without trying to diet, I have lost, or gained, weight.**

| | |
|---|---|
| First Answer | ☐ |
| Second Answer | ☒ |
| Third Answer | ☐ |
| Fourth Answer | ☐ |
| Fifth Answer | ☐ |
| Sixth Answer | ☐ |

Add up all your points to obtain a total score

- Not at all = 0
- Just a little – 1 point
- Somewhat = 2 points
- Moderately = 3 points
- Quite a lot = 4 points
- Very much = 5 points

Find your total score on the Interpretation Table below

Score Interpretation

54 and up    Severely Clinically Depressed

36 - 53    Clinically Depressed, Moderate - Severe

22 - 35    Clinically Depressed, Mild - Moderate

18 - 21    Borderline Clinical Depression

10 - 17    Possibly Mildly Depressed

0 - 9   No Depression Likely

SCORE    **39**

Here is a story about a sufferer of panic attacks and how they dealt with this problem. We hope you will read this story and come to understand how people suffering from depression, anxiety and low self esteem can help themselves massively with the realisation that just facing their problems is in itself such a massive positive statement. This statement they should be able to wallow and enjoy a warm glow. They are fully entitled to feel so good about facing up to their problems.

"People who have never experienced a panic attack often judge the anxious person harshly. The outsider has no real comprehension of what is happening to the person experiencing a panic attack and wonders why they fear to do the simplest things.

I know myself that I could not understand how overnight I went from being a confident young man to someone who became anxious of common everyday situations. Going places took on a whole new dimension as I constantly evaluated if being there might trigger a panic attack.

I had to force myself to do very simple things like go to the cinema or driving in traffic. As a man, that type of anxiety really erodes self confidence, as so much of male self esteem comes from being perceived as strong and brave.

...but here I was afraid to queue at the bank!

Today I know better. Through my own journey and all those I have worked with, I know now that anxiety disorders have nothing to do with a person's level of bravery. I know this to be true because I have worked with many people from the bravest professions around. Firemen, policemen and soldiers. All of them are admired by others for their bravery. Some of these individuals would actually prefer to run into a burning building than stay awake at night with a panic attack. That sounds strange but it isn't really. In a burning building they knew what to do and how to handle the situation. During a panic attack they felt powerless and out of control.

What you have to remember is that panic attacks and general anxiety have no relationship to the level of courage an individual has. In fact it has nothing to do with the world out there. It is a problem born out of an internal crisis. It is easy to feel brave and fearless in the world when your internal world feels safe but when you feel those internal walls have been breached by fear, then your confidence is rocked. The danger you fear becomes internal. Your psychic foundations feel vulnerable. That is where the crisis originates. The doubting of your ability to handle the sensations shakes your inner confidence and that is what the fear feeds off. It is a crisis of confidence in your body and mind's ability to handle the stress. This crisis however does not stop the bravery.

People with anxiety actually do the bravest of things. They get up each day and get on with life. Picking themselves up after each and every setback. It does not make headline news but it counts because it is real bravery, true courage. To the untrained eye it does not seem such a big deal to simply drive a long distance, attend church or go shopping. However, for the person with anxiety that experience can be a massive accomplishment, especially if they have tried and failed many times before.

The good news is this bravery does not go unrewarded. Once the person has triumphed over their anxiety problem, they develop an inner strength that the average person never gets to develop. You see, no matter how many brave things you do in the world, if you have not been challenged on an inner level, then you miss out on the opportunity to develop real inner strength.

That is the hidden opportunity anxiety presents to you. It is to become a bigger person than you already are. That is what you take from the challenge of anxiety. It does not matter if you have not reached that point yet. The journey is unique to everyone so do not judge your progress against others. The only thing that matters is that you persist. Persistence will ensure your success."

This is a true story. Although it is written by a person who suffered from anxiety symptoms, it could just as easily have been written by one who suffered from depression. The problem is it can often be similar, and just as debilitating and difficult to treat. The person that does deal with it is entitled to feel proud that they have had the inner strength to get to grips with such difficult problems.

So you see that depression is a very complex illness. No-one really knows for certain what causes depression, and everyone's experience of depression is different.

Depressive disorders come in different types, just as is the case with other illnesses such as heart disease. When a psychiatrist makes a diagnosis of a patient's depressive illness, he or she may use a number of terms such as:-

- bipolar

- clinical

- endogenous

- major

- melancholic

- seasonal affective

- unipolar

These labels confuse many people who do not understand that they can overlap. People with depressive illness may also receive more than one diagnosis since the illness is often linked with other problems, such as alcoholism or other substance abuses, eating disorders and anxiety disorders.

Depression can also categorise in the following manner:-

1. depression originating from a bad or disturbing event in your life

2. depression which appears without apparent cause - the most common

The first type of depression is easier for you to tackle because the cause is known. The first step is to deal with the event that triggered your depression. It may have started as a result of a death, an accident, a divorce or any other type of setback. The second type of depression is more difficult to deal with as the source is unknown. It is the most common form of depression.

Getting proper help for different types of depression begins with a proper diagnosis. There are several different diagnoses for depression, mostly determined by the intensity, duration and specific cause (if known) of the symptoms.

For 20 percent to 35 percent of depressed people, a normal routine is all but impossible. Others have episodes of depression followed by feelings of well-being. Still others have episodes of terrible lows that alternate with inappropriate "highs." Here are some descriptions of the most common forms of depression.

Let us now consider the diagnoses one by one and see what the essential features of each of the type of depression are:-

- Major Depression - Major depression is a problem with mood in which there are severe and long lasting feelings of sadness or related symptoms that get in the way of a person's functioning.

- Dysthymic Disorder - A less severe type of depression. This involves chronic symptoms that do not disable, but keep one from functioning well or from feeling good.

- Cyclothymic Disorder - A milder form of manic depression, characterised by hypomania (a mild form of mania) alternating with mild bouts of depression.

- Bipolar Disorder (also kmown manic-depressive illness ) - This covers all types of Bipolar Disorder, their treatment options, occurence in childhood, diagnosis criteria, etc.

- Unipolar Depression - This lowered mood may vary slightly throughout the day, but the sufferer cannot usually be cheered up. This is the major distinction between simply being unhappy and being clinically depressed.

- Manic Depression - This can be defined as an emotional disorder characterised by changing mood shifts from depression to mania which can sometimes be quite rapid. People who suffer from manic depression have an extremely high rate of suicide.

- Atypical depression

- Psychotic Depression

# DEPRESSION

Approximately 15 percent of people who suffer from major depression also show symptoms of psychotic depression. These symptoms include:-

- auditory hallucinations (hearing voices in one's head)
- visual hallucinations (having visions of people or things)
- delusional thinking

People who suffer from this extreme form of major depression are in need of immediate attention. Because they cannot rationally judge the consequences of their actions, they are in serious danger of killing themselves.

Severity of depression:-

- mild depression
- moderate depression
- severe depression

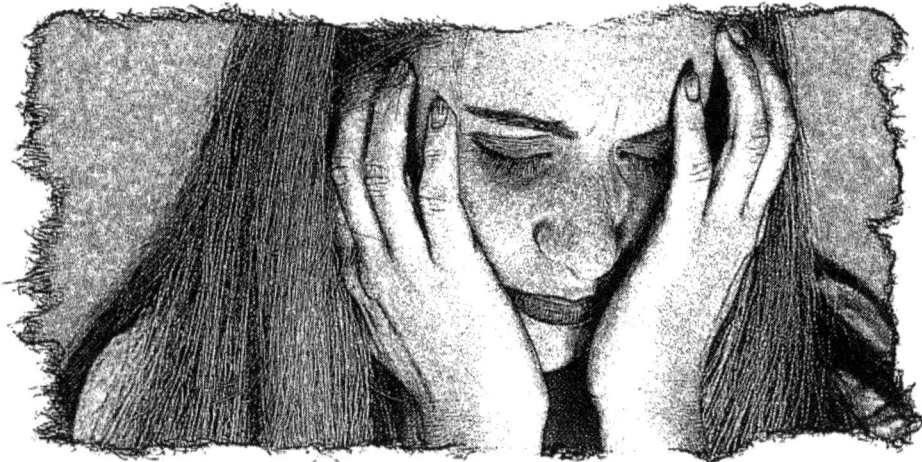

## OTHER DISORDERS

Apart from the types of depression mentioned earlier, there are other disorders featuring various types of depression. Some types of depression have particular symptoms, or are seen in particular situations and age groups, and have special names.

These types of depression may be difficult to identify. They are often similar to other illnesses. In a worst case scenario this may result in the illness going untreated.

It is important to be able to make a diagnosis and start the right treatment in these circumstances.

- Winter depression - Seasonal Affective Disorder (SAD).
- Post Traumatic Stress Disorder - Posttraumatic Stress

Disorder is a complex health condition that can develop in response to a traumatic experience - a life-threatening or extremely distressing situation that causes a person to feel intense fear, horror or a sense of helplessness.

- Postpartum Depression - As the name implies, Postpartum Depression or postnatal depression occurs up to six weeks after a women has given birth.

- Postpartum psychosis

- Neurasthenia

- Puerperal Psychosis

- Premenstrual Dysphoric Disorder (PMDD)

- Neurotic depression

- Masked depression

- Endogenous depression

- Melancholia

- Agitated Depression

- Manic Depressive Disorder

- Manic Depressive Psychosis

- Depressive Disorder NOS

- Dysphoric Mania

## TASKS

Your task at the end of this Chapter 10 is to examine the Activity and Mood Chart, then prepare your own. You may copy or print the example or of course modify this to suit your own need

Please fill in a further Mood Compass as before.

*Try to put your happiness before anyone else's, because you may never have done so in your entire life, if you really think about it, if you are really honest with yourself.*

*Margaret Cho*

**PERSONAL CHART – ACTIVITY AND MOOD CHART**

| TIME | ACTIVITY AND MOOD SCORE OUT OF 10 | ACTIVITY AND MOOD SCORE OUT OF 10 | ACTIVITY AND MOOD SCORE OUT OF 10 | ACTIVITY AND MOOD SCORE OUT OF 10 | ACTIVITY AND MOOD SCORE OUT OF 10 |
|---|---|---|---|---|---|
| 7 – 9 am | | | | | |
| 9 – 12 am | | | | | |
| 12 – 2 pm | | | | | |
| 2 – 5 pm | | | | | |
| 5 – 7 pm | | | | | |
| 7 – 9 pm | | | | | |
| 9 – 11 pm | | | | | |

MENTAL REACTION

MIND

BODY

PHYSICAL REACTION

This is the final chapter, and it is our intention to summarise the kind of things we have tried to show you so that you are able to go forward and deal effectively with your symptoms of low mood, whether it be depression, anxiety or even bipolar related. The methods that we have outlined throughout this book have been field tested extensively and have shown their true worth in the genuine and lasting improvements and relief from symptoms of those who have tried them and put them into practice.

# CHAPTER 11: SUMMARY

# CHAPTER 11: SUMMARY

*Being happy doesn't mean that everything is perfect. It means
that you've decided to look beyond the imperfections.*

*(unknown)*

People with low mood or depressive illnesses do not all experience the same symptoms. The severity, frequency and duration of symptoms will vary depending on the individual's particular illness.

Symptoms include:

- Persistent sad, anxious or "empty" feelings.

- Feelings of hopelessness and/or pessimism.

- Feelings of guilt, worthlessness and/or helplessness.

- Irritability, restlessness.

- Loss of interest in activities or hobbies once pleasurable, including sex.

- Fatigue and decreased energy.

- Difficulty concentrating, remembering details and making decisions.

- Insomnia, early-morning wakefulness, or excessive sleeping.

- Overeating, or appetite loss.

- Thoughts of suicide, suicide attempts.

- Persistent aches or pains, headaches, cramps or digestive problems that do not ease even with treatment.

Depression or low mood has been described as a dysfunction, although this is by no means conclusive. There is a strong school of thought that believes that depression is itself an adaptive defence mechanism, rather than an illness as such. This of course it does not mitigate these severe symptoms experienced by the sufferer. It is merely a label.

The Diagnostic and Statistical Manual of Mental Disorders defines a depressed person as experiencing feelings of sadness, helplessness and hopelessness. In traditional terms feeling depressed is often used as a shorthand term for feeling sad. However, both clinical and nonclinical depression can refer to a much more varied and wider range of symptoms rather than the oversimplistic term of side.

# SUMMARY

So what causes low mood and its related illnesses? It is currently believed that approximately one in six adults suffers from depression at some time during their life. Although depression is not believed to have a single cause, such as certain personality types, there are definitely dramatic events that can trigger the onset of depression such as the death of a close family member. There are also differences in the way depression is generally reported between men and women. Such symptoms as malnutrition, heredity, hormones, seasons, stress, illness, drug and alcohol abuse may present. Insomnia is perhaps one of the commonest symptoms experienced in patients with low mood and depressive illnesses, as many as nine out of ten reporting this problem.

How do we treat low mood and its related illnesses? It would be reasonable to divide treatment into drug and nondrug therapies. As outlined at the beginning of this book we are not intending to go into a discussion of the various drug therapies that are available. There are a great number of manuals that can best inform you of these products and of course you are always well advised to seek a medical professional when looking to take drug therapy as an option. You should bear in mind that drug therapies themselves can divide into two distinct sections.

Firstly there are the manufactured drugs such as Prozac and many other related products that have been produced to relieve depressive symptoms.

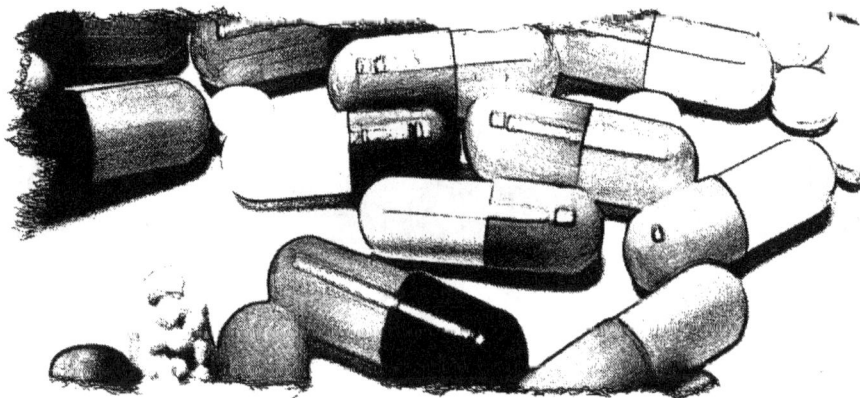

Secondly, there are herbal remedies such as St John's Wort, which has often been reported as being extremely successful in the treatment of depressive illness.

If you are interested in herbal treatments or indeed non-herbal drug treatments there is much information available and you would be well advised to speak to your health professional about these options.

Is low mood or depression a defence mechanism? There has been a significant body of research that suggests depression has adapted people in an evolutionary way, so that a low mood is a defence mechanism which allows a person to cope with and deal with certain situations such as danger and loss. The theory is that low mood works by inhibiting certain actions, for example

189

shutting off the extremes of reaction and allowing the dramatic or other event to take its course. On the other hand, if depression is an illness or dysfunction this phenomenon is less likely, though not impossible in certain cases.

Of course as we stated earlier in certain dramatic and tragic events the onset of low mood is inevitable, or virtually inevitable. Divorce, death of a child or spouse, and even the loss of a cherished job or career or business setback are all events that can bring on low mood. There is some evidence to support this, in that people tend to be most at risk from depression during their peak years.

Let us summarise what we have learned and covered during the preceding ten chapters so that we are able to formulate our own personal action plan to recover from the low mood symptoms that are preventing us from enjoying the fullest quality-of-life.

In Chapter 1 we introduced you to the four mood compass. This is a proven device that has enabled people to understand and get to grips with the symptoms of low mood from which they are suffering and to see them in a very visual manner that enables them to understand what they are going through and monitor and plan their progress of recovery.

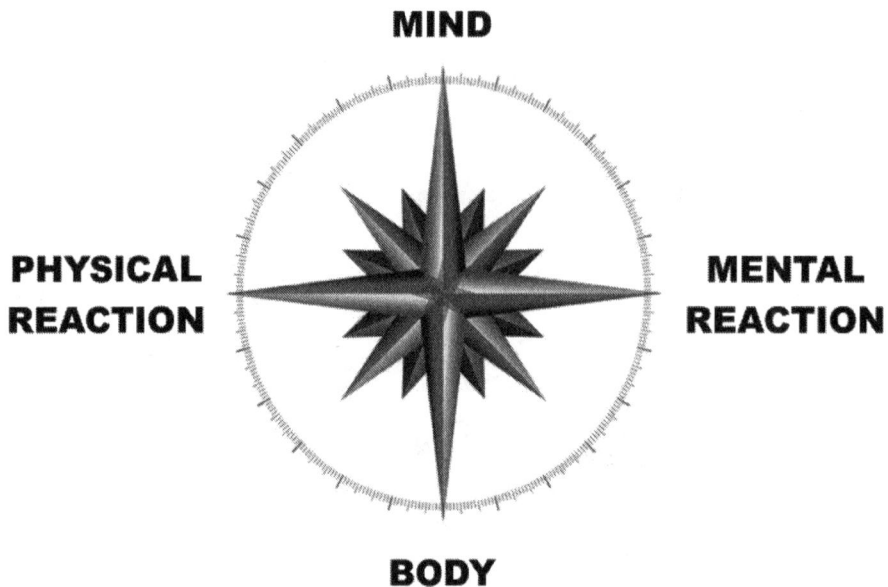

**MIND**

**PHYSICAL
REACTION**

**MENTAL
REACTION**

**BODY**

We introduced you to three of the people who have been treated using the methods outlined in this book, Jane, Susan and Tony. We hope that it is clear that low mood is something that is suffered by a wide variety of people in a wide variety of situations. It could be men or women, young or old, people that have recently suffered bereavement or last or people for whom the dark cloud of low mood has suddenly descended for no obvious or apparent reason. Do we need really to understand the reason for low mood? It is debatable, and we have certainly tried to explain and clarify many of the reasons why this illness occurs. However, we are convinced, and hope you will agree, that by far the

MENTAL REACTION

MIND

PHYSICAL REACTION

BODY

most important factor is to elevate low mood and returned the sufferer's life to happiness and fulfillment.

Therefore we have devised a continuing programme of mood development. In Chapter 1 we asked you to draw a simple minded compass and fill it in with those aspects of your mood that you feel are most important to you. We also are asked to think about your past life and to consider the degree to which you have suffered from low mood previously, and to also write these things down. The mind compass is an important tool for you to use in the cause of your recovery and what we would suggest now is:-

## TASK

Fill in a mood compass that describes your mood at the end of this book. Then compare this compass with the one that you prepared at the very end of Chapter 1. Put these sheets into a ring binder with the most recent sheet to the front. Make a note in your diary, planner or notice board in the kitchen that you will complete a mood compass on a weekly basis on the same day each week.

In Chapter 2 we further examined the three subjects, Jane, Susan and Tony to see how events in their lives had brought on the onset of low mood related problems. We introduced you to the concept of perception. What is clear for many mood sufferers is that the reason for their suffering so badly is, not so much that they have problems that are very real but, that they have problems they perceive in a way that is the opposite from the way non-sufferers would perceive them. (Of course, in cases such as bereavement and perhaps very severe illness the reason is clear and obvious). We asked you to write a list of the kinds of difficulties you are currently experiencing that you feel are causing you to suffer, and the way you perceive these difficulties are harming or causing you to suffer in each case. Then, for each difficulty how this could perhaps be perceived in a different way. The fundamental idea is that some things do happen that you cannot prevent, that you can mitigate the damage and suffering they caused mainly by perceiving them in a different way. A simple example of this would be the loss of a job, which could be perceived as a tragic loss in itself or alternatively as an opportunity to start a much more interesting and rewarding career.

In Chapter 3 we began to look at the components that make up mood by asking the question "what is mood?" We looked further and deeper into our example subjects to get a wider view of why they were suffering the problems that they were. Hopefully we were able to illustrate how complex these problems could be during their development. At the same time we would reiterate that while it is important to understand something of the problems you are suffering, in is substantially more important to work on dealing with and resolving the problem. We introduced you to the concept of making a list of the moods and feelings that you experienced the previous day, what triggered this feeling and how you actually felt both physically and mentally or emotionally about this event. This is an important exercise that will help with the question of how you perceive events that occur in your life and how to perhaps alter your perception in a way that will serve the best, or at least substantially better than previously.

In chapter 4 we introduced the concept of a mood diary, where you were able to more extensively keep a record of the difficulties you were suffering. Keeping a mood diary is a vital part of recovering from symptoms of low mood

# SUMMARY

and we cannot overemphasise the importance of doing this. If you have not already, please doubt now. We also looked at the effect of exercise on mood, although it is dealt with in a later chapter the point was that the most basic simple exercise cannot fail to have a positive effect on the symptoms of low mood. Again, if you have not started a simple exercise programme now is the time to begin, at least do something that will improve your overall fitness even if it is a very gentle and basic to begin with.

In Chapter 5 we examined the difficulties low mood sufferers can experience with automatic thoughts. Automatic thoughts are a simple mental response to a certain stimulus. It is by no means uncommon for low mood sufferers to have automatic thoughts that areunhelpful and bound to increase or worsen their symptoms. Going back to the example of the person who loses their job, the automatic thought from a person who does not suffer from low mood is more likely to be one of optimism at the chance of increasing the richness and variety of their career. The low mood sufferer is far more likely to see the loss of their job as something dark and dreadful that can only lead to chaos and disaster. The technical term for this kind of thinking is Cognitive Distortion, where your core beliefs are inclined to push your thinking in a certain direction. This is a direction certain to only make a bad situation considerably worse. We therefore introduced the concept of the thought monitoring chart so that you would be able to monitor your automatic thoughts and core beliefs. The reason is that when you see your thinking on paper the obvious damage you are causing to yourself that by cognitive distortion is very clear. If you have not already begun working on your thought monitoring chart we would suggest that you re-read Chapter 5 and begin writing out your first chart.

In Chapter 6 we took a more extensive look at exercise and also introduced the concept of nutrition. There is absolutely no doubt whatsoever that any form of gentle exercise will mitigate the symptoms of low mood. For sufferers, the concept of developing and keeping to their gentle programme of regular exercise is absolutely vital if they are to recover good health amd a positive prognosis for the future. We encouraged you to develop your own exercise programme and keep a chart of your progress. There is also the question of nutrition. Without going into the arguments over junk and processed food versus fresh food, there is absolutely no doubt that the healthier your diet the better chance you have of avoiding the worst symptoms of low mood. Although of course merely eating a healthy diet is not in itself sufficient to prevent a low mood in its entirety. It is certain that if you follow the steps of introducing a gentle exercise regime into your lifestyle, together with working to improve the quality of your diet, your symptoms will be mitigated. We introduced you to the concept of making a weight chart to monitor your weight. Also to

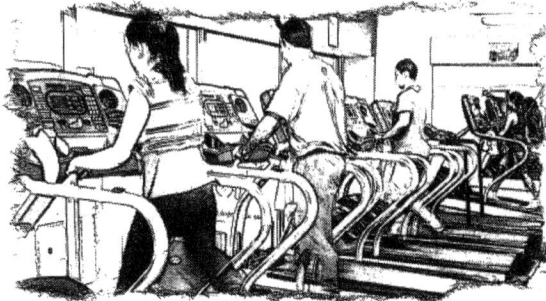

193

complete a similar chart to monitor your nutrition, so that you are able to keep an eye on what you are eating. Having a visual record encourages you to make adjustments and improvements were necessary.

In Chapter 7 we looked further into the concept of your re-examining your thoughts. So that where an event occurs that, is not necessarily one that need not have a negative impact on your mood, you do not unconsciously allow it to have this very effect. This undermining and exacerbating the symptoms you are suffering. It is by no means uncommon to come across the subject of positive thinking. However, this is not entirely a simple process where a person can repeat certain affirmations such as "I feel like a wonderful person" or "I feel that I have a wonderful and golden future ahead of me". Keeping it all in your head is not a good way to a deal with your problems. You need to both write down what has happened and how you have responded to it, together with the various options that would h ave a more beneficial effect on your mood. You also need to take action, physical action, that will itself underpin your recovery. We looked at a mood check chart, which is a simple chart you could use when you feel it is necessary to re-examine and re-evaluate an event in your life that you feel is causing you difficulties. If you have not yet made your own mood check charts we suggest that you do so and begin using them, at this stage on an ad hoc basis will be fine.

In Chapter 8 we introduced the concept of "do something different". Put quite simply, if the response is that you have had so far to stimuli and events that occur in your life have had an effect that is more negative than positive and have caused you to suffer from low mood related symptoms. Clearly you need to approach these stimuli and events in a different way. Frequently it is a matter of taking a chance. A prime example of this was where we looked at the difficulties Tony was having at work with his colleagues, who he thought were seeing him in a very unfavourable light. It was almost certain that the problem was something that Tony had virtually invented, without any real evidence of it being true. Once he was able to visualise the problem, by seeing it on paper, he was able to determine that the best option was to take a chance and attempt to be more sociable with these people. This is exactly what he did in fact do and, not unsurprisingly, the outcome was very favourable. This then enabled him to have a considerably more fulfilling relationship at work, without the enervating effects of feeling despised by his peers. Whilst this did not solve all of Tony's problems at a stroke, let alone his cocaine habit, it was a strong start on the road to recovery. How you respond to situations is vitally important,and generating appropriate responses, as opposed to negative and inappropriate responses, will help you to recover from low mood just as it helped Tony. In order to visualise how you respond to events and how appropriate otherwise this response is, we suggested that you made out your own response chart at the end of chapter 8. If you have not done so, we suggest you do this before proceeding further.

In chapter 9 we examined the problems of low self esteem and the harmful effects it can have on virtually anybody. The causes of low self-esteem are many and varied and can often begin in early childhood. We outlined many of the causes of this complex problem, together with strategies for resolving these issues by changing your interpretation of yourself and the way you act to other people. We urged you to challenge your core beliefs by keeping a record of these core beliefs as they become apparent when certain events crop up. You

# SUMMARY

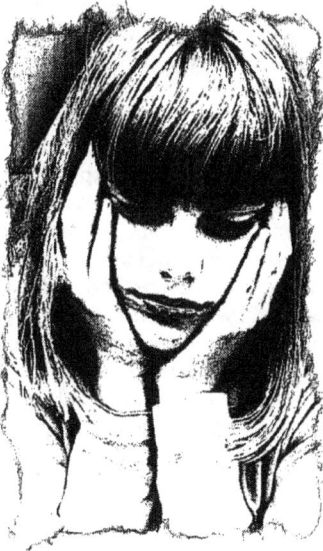

then are required to challenge your core beliefs and examine how they could possibly be flawed, further how you could modify them in such a way that it will benefit you and help lift your mood. Again, if you have not done so already, we suggest that you make out your own core belief challenge charts and begin using them, together with the summaries which will give you a quick visual indication of the progress you are making and what work you need to do in this particular area.

In Chapter 10 we took a longer and deeper look at the whole area of depression, including a questionnaire that serves to diagnose the problem. It is extremely difficult to make a confirmed diagnosis of depression, certainly in a subjective sense. However, the depression questionnaire can be extremely valuable in giving new trends and indicators about yourself, especially if you make it a habit to regularly fill in one of these questionnaires, perhaps on a weekly or even monthly basis. In this way you will have a simple and straightforward record of your mood, either improving or otherwise. If you have not already done so please make out your own questionnaire and pencil in a regular weekly or monthly slot to carry out this process.

Any study of low mood, depression, bipolar disorder, anxiety or related symptoms will frequently come back to the nature or nurture question. There is growing evidence for the importance of genetic factors in clinical depression and depressed mood. Depression can appear to be related to disruptions in the circadian rhythm, or human biological clock.

Major depression may also be caused in part by an overactive Hypothalamic-Pituitary-Adrenal Axis (HPA Axis) that is similar to the neuro-endocrine response to stress. Investigations reveal increased levels of the hormone Cortisol, enlarged pituitary and adrenal glands, and a blunted circadian rhythm. Over secretion of the Corticotropin-releasing hormone from the Hypothalamus is thought to drive this, and is implicated in the cognitive and arousal symptoms. The REM stage of sleep in which dreaming occurs tends to be especially quick to arrive, and especially intense, in depressed people. Although the precise relationship between sleep and depression is mysterious, the relationship appears to be particularly strong among those whose depressive episodes are not precipitated by stress. In such cases, patients may be especially unaffected by therapeutic intervention.

The hormone Oestrogen has been implicated in depressive disorders due to the increase in risk of depressive episodes after puberty, the antenatal period and reduced levels after the menopause. Conversely, the premenstrual and postpartum periods of low Oestrogen levels are also associated with increased risk. The use of Oestrogen has been under researched, although some small trials show promise in its use to prevent or treat depression. The evidence for its effectiveness is not strong. Oestrogen Replacement Therapy has been shown to be beneficial in improving mood in Perimenopause, but it is unclear if it is merely the menopausal symptoms that are being reversed.

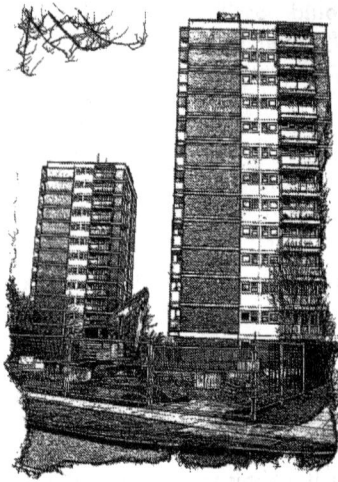

Social depravation, discriminative behaviour towards an individual occurring either explicitly or implicitly (i.e. the director is unaware of their negative behaviour towards the receiver), peer pressure whether implicit (i.e. a natural attempt to conform to social standards, or to compete with social pressure)) or explicit and de-synchronised social interaction primarily act as a social stimulus for depression. The absence of social synchronisation may occur due to an imbalance between independence and external interaction (i.e.socialising) with their environment. Independence would thus be an individual synchronising with their internal mechanisms, causing them to develop extravagant abilities, abnormal academia (depending on age) or abilities to achieve excessive results in challenges of various subjects. A synchronisation period may result in the individual losing their independence and ability to socialise.

Alternative social stimuli for depression may present as requirements for relationships. An individual may find peer pressure directed towards a need for a relationship with either sex. Furthermore, an evolutionary conflict may occur between a social environment. An individual may lack the ability, or refuse, to synchronise with their social environment. Also with additional pressure to sustain a relationship, a conflict may transpire thereby inadvertently causing depression.

Various aspects of personality and its development are integral in the occurrence and persistence of depression. Although episodes are strongly linked to adverse events, how a person copes with stress also plays a role. Low self-esteem, learned helplessness and distorted thinking are related to depression. Depression may also be connected to feelings of religious alienation. Conversely, depression is less likely to occur among those with high levels of religious involvement. It is not always clear which factors are causes or effects of depression, but in any case depressed people who are able to make corrections in their thinking patterns often show improved mood and self-esteem.

Poverty and social isolation are associated with increased risk of psychiatric problems in general. A study in Providence, Rhode Island followed children from birth. It found that family disruption and low socioeconomic status in early childhood were linked to an increased risk of major depression in later life. This was noted to be independent of later adult social status and related to various social inequalities and the consequences of which may be more severe for women. Childhood emotional, physical, sexual abuse or neglect are also associated with increased risk of developing depressive disorders later in life. Disturbances in family functioning, such as parental (particularly maternal) depression, severe marital conflict or divorce, death of a parent or other disturbances in parenting are additional risk factors.

In adulthood stressful life events are strongly associated with the onset of major depressive episodes. A first episode is more likely to be immediately preceded by stressful life events than are recurrent ones. The relationship

# SUMMARY

between stressful life events and social support has been a matter of some debate. Perhaps the lack of social support only increases the likelihood that life stress will lead to depression. More likely, however, the absence of social support constitutes a form of strain that provokes depression directly. There is evidence that neighborhood social disorder, for example, due to crime or illicit drugs, is a risk factor. Alternatively a high neighbourhood socio-economic status, with better amenities, is a protective factor. Adverse workplace conditions, particularly demanding jobs with little scope for decision-making, are associated with depression.

In conclusion, we would state that whilst there is considerable worth and importance in understanding the reasons and causes of low mood and the related illnesses that accompany this phenomenon, it is more important by far to actually come to grips with the problem as it affects you. It is equally important to understand that there is no magic bullet. No single drug, herb or therapy, discussion group or advice is likely of itself to resolve your problems. The only realistic approach to complete relief from your symptoms is a genuinely holistic approach. We hope and trust that in this book we have given you sufficient tools and insights to go forward in the process of relieving your symptoms and ridding yourself of low mood for evermore.

*The reason people find it so hard to be happy is that they always see the past better than it was, the present worse than it is, and the future less resolved than it will be*

*Marcel Pagnol*

# APPENDIX I  UK ADDRESSES

# APPENDIX I UK ADDRESSES

Depression Alliance

35 Westminster Bridge Road,

London SE1 7JB

Tel: 020 7633 0557

e-mail: information@depressionalliance.org

www.depressionalliance.org


Equality & Human Rights Commission

Freepost MID 02164,

Stratford-upon-Avon CV37 9BR

Tel: 08457 622 633

www.equalityhumanrights.com


Mental Health Foundation

83 Victoria Street,

London SW1H 0HW

Tel: 020 7802 0300

e-mail: mhf@mhf.org.uk

www.mentalhealth.org.uk

www.connects.org.uk

# APPENDIX I UK ADDRESSES

Mental Health Media

The Resource Centre,

356 Holloway Road,

London N7 6PA

Tel: 020 7700 8171

e-mail: info@mhmedia.com

www.mhmedia.com


Mind

Granta House,

15-19 Broadway,

London E15 4BQ

Tel: 020 8519 2122

Fax: 020 8522 1725

e-mail: info@mind.org.uk

www.mind.org.uk


National Institute for Adult & Continuing Education NIACE/NIMHE Partnership

Renaissance House

20 Princess Road West

Leicester

LE1 6TP

United Kingdom

Tel: 0116 204 4200

e-mail: kathryn.james@niace.org.uk

www.niace.org.uk


National Institute for Mental Health England (NIMHE)

Blenheim House

West One

Duncombe Street

Leeds LS1 4Pl

Tel: 0113 254 5000

www.nimhe.csip.org.uk & Knowledge Community


NIMHE South West

Mallard Court

Express Park

Bristol Road

Bridgwater TA6 4RN

Tel: 01278 432002

www.nimhe.csip.org.uk


Rethink

30 Tabernacle Street,

London EC2A 4DD

Tel: 020 7330 9100

e-mail: info@rethink.org

www.rethink.org


Sainsbury Centre for Mental Health

134 Borough High Street,

London SE1 1LB

Tel: 020 7403 8790

Fax: 020 7403 9482

e-mail: contact@scmh.org.uk

www.scmh.org.uk


Sane

1st Floor, Cityside House,

## APPENDIX I UK ADDRESSES

40 Adler Street,

London E1 1EE

Tel: 020 7375 1002

Helpline: 0845 767 8000

e-mail: london@sane.org.uk

www.sane.org.uk


Together (formerly MACA)

25 Bedford Square,

London WC1B 3HW

Tel: 020 7436 6194

e-mail: info@together-uk.org

www.together-uk.org

# APPENDIX II US ADDRESSES

# APPENDIX II US ADDRESSES

Teen Suicide Hotline: (1-800-784-2433)

1-800-SUICIDE

http://www.yellowribbon.org


Suicide Hotline: 1-800-SUICIDE

(1-800-784-2433)


Depression Hotline: 630-482-9696


American Psychiatric Association (APA)

1000 Wilson Boulevard, Suite 1825

Arlington, VA 22209-3901

Phone: 703-907-7300

http://www.psych.org/index.cfm


American Psychological Association

750 1st Street, NE

Washington, DC 20002-4242

Phone: 202-336-5510

TollFree: 1-800-374-2721

http://www.apa.org

# APPENDIX I US ADDRESSES

Depression and Bipolar Support Alliance (DBSA)

730 N. Franklin Street, Suite 501

Chicago, IL 60610-7224

Phone: 312-642-0049

Fax: 312-642-7243

http://www.DBSAlliance.org


Depression and Related Affective Disorders Association (DRADA)

2330 West Joppa Road, Suite 100

Lutherville, MD 21093

Phone: 410-583-2919

Email: drada@jhmi.edu

http://www.drada.org


National Alllance for Research on Schizophrenia and Depression (NARSAD)

60 Cutter Mill Road, Suite 404

Great Neck, NY 11021

Phone: 516-829-0091

TollFree: 800-829-8289

Email: info@narsad.org

http://www.narsad.org


National Foundation for Depressive Illness, Inc. (NAFDI)

PO Box 2257

New York, NY 10116

TollFree: 800-239-1265

http://www.depression.org

# GLOSSARY

# GLOSSARY

## A

abreaction An emotional release or discharge after recalling a painful experience that has been repressed because it was not consciously tolerable. Often the release is surprising to the individual experiencing it because of it's intensity and the circumstances surrounding its onset. A therapeutic effect sometimes occurs through partial or repeated discharge of the painful affect.

abstract attitude (categorical attitude) This is a type of thinking that includes voluntarily shifting one's mind set from a specific aspect of a situation to the general aspect; It involves keeping in mind different simultaneous aspects of a situation while grasping the essentials of the situation. It can involve breaking a situation down into its parts and isolating them voluntarily; planning ahead ideationally; and/or thinking or performing symbolically. A characteristic of many psychiatric disorders is the person's inability to assume the abstract attitude or to shift readily from the concrete to the abstract and back again as demanded by circumstances.

abulia A lack of will or motivation which is often expressed as inability to make decisions or set goals. Often, the reduction in impulse to action and thought is coupled with an indifference or lack of concern about the consequences of action.

acalculia The loss of a previously possessed ability to engage in arithmetic calculation.

acculturation difficulty A problem stemming from an inability to appropriately adapt to a different culture or environment. The problem is not based on any coexisting mental disorder.

acetylcholine A neurotransmitter in the brain, which helps to regulate memory, and in the peripheral nervous system, where it affects the actions of skeletal and smooth muscle.

acting out This is the process of expressing unconscious emotional conflicts or feelings via actions rather than words. The person is not consciously aware of the meaning or etiology of such acts. Acting out may be harmful or, in controlled situations, therapeutic (e.g., children's play therapy).

actualization The realization of one's full potential - intellectual, psychological, physical, etc.

adiadochokinesia The inability to perform rapid alternating movements of one or more of the extremities. This task is sometimes requested by physicians of patients during physical examinations to determine if there exists neurological problems.

adrenergic This refers to neuronal or neurologic activity caused by neurotransmitters such as epinephrine, norepinephrine, and dopamine.

affect This word is used to described observable behavior that represents the expression of a subjectively experienced feeling state (emotion). Common examples of affect are sadness, fear, joy, and anger. The normal range of expressed affect varies considerably between different cultures and even within the same culture. Types of affect include: euthymic, irritable, constricted; blunted; flat; inappropriate, and labile.

affective disorders Refers to disorders of mood. Examples would include Major Depressive Disorder, Dysthymia, Depressive Disorder, N.O.S., Adjustment Disorder with Depressed Mood, Bipolar Disorder...

age-associated memory impairment (AAMI) The mild disturbance in memory function that occurs normally with aging; benign senescent forgetfulness. Such lapses in memory are lately humorously referred to as representing "a senior moment".

agitation (psychomotor agitation) Excessive motor activity that accompanies and is associated with a feeling of inner tension. The activity is usually nonproductive and repetitious and consists of such behavior as pacing, fidgeting, wringing of the hands, pulling of clothes, and inability to sit still.

agnosia Failure to recognize or identify objects despite intact sensory function; This may be seen in dementia of various types. An example would be the failure of someone to recognize a paper clip placed in their hand while keeping their eyes closed.

agonist medication A chemical entity that is not naturally occuring within the body which acts upon a receptor and is capable of producing the maximal effect that can be produced by stimulating that receptor. A partial agonist is capable only of producing less than the maximal effect even when given in a concentration sufficient to bind with all available receptors.

agonist/antagonist medication A chemical entity that is not naturally occuring within the body which acts on a family of receptors (such as mu, delta, and kappa opiate receptors) in such a fashion that it is an agonist or partial agonist on one type of receptor while at the same time it is also an antagonist on another different receptor.

agoraphobia Anxiety about being in places or situations in which escape might be difficut or embarrassing or in which help may not be available should a panic attack occur. The fears typically relate to venturing into the open, of leaving the familiar setting of one's home, or of being in a crowd, standing in line, or traveling in a car or train. Although agoraphobia usually occurs as a part of panic disorder, agoraphobia without a history of panic disorder has been described as also occuring without other disorders.

agraphia The loss of a pre-existing ability to express one's self through the act of writing.

akathisia Complaints of restlessness accompanied by movements such as fidgeting of the legs, rocking from foot to foot, pacing, or inability to sit or stand. Symptoms can develop within a few weeks of starting or raising the dose of traditional neuroleptic medications or of reducing the dose of medication used to treat extrapyramidal symptoms. akathisia is a state of motor restlessness ranging from a feeling of inner disquiet to inability to sit still or lie quietly.

akinesia A state of motor inhibition or reduced voluntary movement.

akinetic mutism A state of apparent alertness with following eye movements but no speech or voluntary motor responses.

alexia Loss of a previously intact ability to grasp the meaning of written or printed words and sentences.

alexithymia A disturbance in affective and cognitive function that can be present in an assortment of diagnostic entities. Is common in psychosomatic disorders, addictive disorders, and posttraumatic stress disorder. The chief manifestations are difficulty in describing or recognizing one's own emotions, a limited fantasy life, and general constriction in affective life.

algophobia Fear of pain.

alienation The estrangement felt in a setting one views as foreign, unpredictable, or unacceptable. For example, in depersonalization phenomena, feelings of unreality or strangeness produce a sense of alienation from one's self or environment.

alloplastic Referring to adaptation by means of altering the external environment. This can be contrasted to autoplastic, which refers to the alteration of one's own behavior and responses.

alogia An impoverishment in thinking that is inferred from observing speech and language behavior. There may be brief and concrete replies to questions and restriction in the amount of spontaneous speech (poverty of speech). Sometimes the speech is adequate in amount but conveys little information because it is overconcrete, overabstract, repetitive, or stereotyped (poverty of content).

ambivalence The coexistence of contradictory emotions, attitudes, ideas, or desires with respect to a particular person, object, or situation. Ordinarily, the ambivalence is not fully conscious and suggests psychopathology only when present in an extreme form.

amentia Subnormal development of the mind, with particular reference to intellectual capacities; a type of severe mental retardation.

amimia A disorder of language characterized by an inability to make gestures or to understand the significance of gestures.

amines Organic compounds containing the amino group. Amines such as epinephrine and norepinephrine are significant because they function as neurotransmitters.

amnesia Loss of memory. Types of amnesia include: anterograde Loss of memory of events that occur after the onset of the etiological condition or agent. retrograde Loss of memory of events that occurred before the onset of the etiological condition or agent.

amok A culture specific syndrome from Malay involving acute indiscriminate homicidal mania .

amygdala This is a structure of the brain which is part of the basal ganglia located on the roof of the temporal horn of the lateral ventricle at the inferior end of the caudate nucleus. It is a structure in the forebrain that is an important component of the limbic system.

amyloid Any one of various complex proteins that are deposited in tissues in different disease processes. These proteins have an affinity for Congo red dye. In neuropsychiatry, of particular interest are the beta-amyloid (A4) protein, which is the major component of the characteristic senile plaques of Alzheimer's disease, and the amyloid precursor protein (APP).

anaclitic In psychoanalytic terminology, dependence of the infant on the mother or mother substitute for a sense of well-being. This is considered normal behavior in childhood, but pathologic in later years.

anal stage The period of pregenital psychosexual development, usually from 1 to 3 years, in which the child has particular interest and concern with the process of defecation and the sensations connected with the anus. The pleasurable part of the experience is termed anal eroticism.

anamnesis The developmental history of a patient and of his or her illness, especially recollections.

anankastic personality Synonym for obsessive-compulsive personality.

androgyny A combination of male and female characteristics in one person.

anhedonia Inability to experience pleasure from activities that usually produce pleasurable feelings. Contrast with hedonism.

anima In Jungian psychology, a person's inner being as opposed to the character or persona presented to the world. Further, the anima may be the more feminine "soul" or inner self of a man, and the animus the more masculine soul of a woman.

anomie Apathy, alienation, and personal distress resulting from the loss of goals previously valued. Emile Durkheim popularized this term when he listed it as a principal reason for suicide.

anosognosia The apparent unawareness of or failure to recognize one's own functional defect (e.g., hemiplegia, hemianopsia).

antagonist medication A chemical entity that is not naturally occuring within the body which occupies a receptor, produces no physiologic effects, and prevents endogenous and exogenous chemicals from producing an effect on that receptor.

anxiety The apprehensive anticipation of future danger or misfortune accompanied by a feeling of dysphoria or somatic symptoms of tension. The focus of anticipated danger may be internal or external. Anxiety is often distinguished from fear in that fear is a more appropriate word to use when there exists threat or danger in the real world. Anxiety is reflective more of a threat that is not apparent or imminent in the real world, at least not to the experienced degree.

apathy Lack of feeling, emotion, interest, or concern.

aphasia An impairment in the understanding or transmission of ideas by language in any of its forms--reading, writing, or speaking--that is due to injury or disease of the brain centers involved in language.

anomic or amnestic aphasia Loss of the ability to name objects.

aphonia An inability to produce speech sounds that require the use of the larynx that is not due to a lesion in the central nervous system.

apperception Perception as modified and enhanced by one's own emotions, memories, and biases.

apraxia Inability to carry out previously learned skilled motor activities despite intact comprehension and motor function; this may be seen in dementia.

assimilation A Piagetian term describing a person's ability to comprehend and integrate new experiences.

astereognosis Inability to recognize familiar objects by touch that cannot be explained by a defect of elementary tactile sensation.

ataxia Partial or complete loss of coordination of voluntary muscular movement.

attention The ability to focus in a sustained manner on a particular stimulus or activity. A disturbance in attention may be manifested by easy distractibility or difficulty in finishing tasks or in concentrating on work

auditory hallucination A hallucination involving the perception of sound, most commonly of voices. Some clinicians and investigators would not include those experiences perceived as coming from inside the head and would instead limit the concept of true auditory hallucinations to those sounds whose source is perceived as being external.

aura A premonitory, subjective brief sensation (e.g., a flash of light) that warns of an impending headache or convulsion. The nature of the sensation depends on the brain area in which the attack begins. Seen in migraine and epilepsy.

autoeroticism Sensual self-gratification. Characteristic of, but not limited to, an early stage of emotional development. Includes satisfactions derived from genital play, masturbation, fantasy, and oral, anal, and visual sources.

automatism Automatic and apparently undirected nonpurposeful behavior that is not consciously controlled. Seen in psychomotor epilepsy.

autoplastic Referring to adaptation by changing the self.

autotopagnosia Inability to localize and name the parts of one's own body.

finger agnosia would be autotopagnosia restricted to the fingers.

avolition An inability to initiate and persist in goal-directed activities. When severe enough to be considered pathological, avolition is pervasive and prevents the person from completing many different types of activities (e.g., work, intellectual pursuits, self-care).

**B**

basal gangliaClusters of neurons located deep in the brain; they include the caudate nucleus and the putamen (corpus striatum), the globus pallidus, the subthalamic nucleus, and the substantia nigra. The basal ganglia appear to be involved in higher-order aspects of motor control, such as planning and execution of complex motor activity and the speed of movements. Lesions of the basal ganglia produce various types of involuntary movements such as athetosis, chorea, dystonia, and tremor. The basal ganglia are involved also in the pathophysiology of Parkinson's disease, Huntington's disease, and tardive dyskinesia. The internal capsule, containing all the fibers that ascend to or descend from the cortex, runs through the basal ganglia and separates them from the thalamus.

bestiality Zoophilia; sexual relations between a human being and an animal. See also paraphilia.

beta-blocker An agent that inhibits the action of beta-adrenergic receptors, which modulate cardiac functions, respiratory functions, and the dilation of blood vessels. Beta-blockers are of value in the treatment of hypertension, cardiac arrhythmias, and migraine. In psychiatry, they have been used in the treatment of aggression and violence, anxiety-related tremors and lithium-induced tremors, neuroleptic-induced akathisia, social phobias, panic states, and alcohol withdrawal.

bizarre delusion A delusion that involves a phenomenon that the person's culture would regard as totally implausible.

blind spot Visual scotoma, a circumscribed area of blindness or impaired vision in the visual field; by extension, an area of the personality of which the subject is unaware, typically because recognition of this area would cause painful emotions.

blocking A sudden obstruction or interruption in spontaneous flow of thinking or speaking, perceived as an absence or deprivation of thought.

blunted affect An affect type that represents significant reduction in the intensity of emotional expression

body image One's sense of the self and one's body.

bradykinesia Neurologic condition characterized by a generalized slowness of motor activity.

Broca's aphasia Loss of the ability to comprehend language coupled with production of inappropriate language.

bruxism Grinding of the teeth, occurs unconsciously while awake or during stage 2 sleep. May be secondary to anxiety, tension, or dental problems.

## C

Capgras' syndrome The delusion that others, or the self, have been replaced by imposters. It typically follows the development of negative feelings toward the other person that the subject cannot accept and attributes, instead, to the imposter. The syndrome has been reported in paranoid schizophrenia and, even more frequently, in organic brain disease.

catalepsy Waxy flexibility--rigid maintenance of a body position over an extended period of time.

cataplexy Episodes of sudden bilateral loss of muscle tone resulting in the individual collapsing, often in association with intense emotions such as laughter, anger, fear, or surprise.

catatonic behavior Marked motor abnormalities including motoric immobility (i.e., catalepsy or stupor), certain types of excessive motor activity (apparently purposeless agitation not influenced by external stimuli), extreme negativism (apparent motiveless resistance to instructions or attempts to be moved) or mutism, posturing or stereotyped movements, and echolalia or echopraxia

catharsis The healthful (therapeutic) release of ideas through "talking out" conscious material accompanied by an appropriate emotional reaction. Also, the release into awareness of repressed ("forgotten") material from the unconscious. See also repression.

cathexis Attachment, conscious or unconscious, of emotional feeling and significance to an idea, an object, or, most commonly, a person.

causalgia A sensation of intense pain of either organic or psychological origin.

cerea flexibilitas The "waxy flexibility" often present in catatonic schizophrenia in which the patient's arm or leg remains in the position in which it is placed.

circumstantiality Pattern of speech that is indirect and delayed in reaching its goal because of excessive or irrelevant detail or parenthetical remarks. The speaker does not lose the point, as is characteristic of loosening of associations, and clauses remain logically connected, but to the listener it seems that the end will never be reached.

clanging A type of thinking in which the sound of a word, rather than its meaning, gives the direction to subsequent associations.

climacteric Menopausal period in women. Sometimes used to refer to the corresponding age period in men. Also called involutional period.

cognitive Pertaining to thoughts or thinking. Cognitive disorders are disorders of thinking, for example, schizophrenia.

comorbidity The simultaneous appearance of two or more illnesses, such as the co-occurrence of schizophrenia and substance abuse or of alcohol dependence and depression. The association may reflect a causal relationship between one disorder and another or an underlying vulnerability to both disorders. Also, the appearance of the illnesses may be unrelated to any common etiology or vulnerability.

compensation A defense mechanism, operating unconsciously, by which one attempts to make up for real or fancied deficiencies. Also a conscious process in which one strives to make up for real or imagined defects of physique, performance skills, or psychological attributes. The two types frequently merge. See also overcompensation.

compulsion Repetitive ritualistic behavior such as hand washing or ordering or a mental act such as praying or repeating words silently that aims to prevent or reduce distress or prevent some dreaded event or situation. The person feels driven to perform such actions in response to an obsession or according to rules that must be applied rigidly, even though the behaviors are recognized to be excessive or unreasonable.

conative Pertains to one's basic strivings as expressed in behavior and actions

concrete thinking Thinking characterized by immediate experience, rather than abstractions. It may occur as a primary, developmental defect, or it may develop secondary to organic brain disease or schizophrenia.

condensation A psychological process, often present in dreams, in which two or more concepts are fused so that a single symbol represents the multiple components.

confabulation Fabrication of stories in response to questions about situations or events that are not recalled.

confrontation A communication that deliberately pressures or invites another to self-examine some aspect of behavior in which there is a discrepancy between self-reported and observed behavior.

constricted affect Affect type that represents mild reduction in the range and intensity of emotional expression.

constructional apraxia An acquired difficulty in drawing two-dimensional objects or forms, or in producing or copying three-dimensional arrangements of forms or shapes.

contingency reinforcement In operant or instrumental conditioning, ensuring that desired behavior is followed by positive consequences and that undesired behavior is not rewarded.

conversion A defense mechanism, operating unconsciously, by which intrapsychic conflicts that would otherwise give rise to anxiety are instead given symbolic external expression. The repressed ideas or impulses, and the psychological defenses against them, are converted into a variety of somatic symptoms. These may include such symptoms as paralysis, pain, or loss of sensory function.

coping mechanisms Ways of adjusting to environmental stress without altering one's goals or purposes; includes both conscious and unconscious mechanisms.

coprophagia Eating of filth or feces.

counterphobia Deliberately seeking out and exposing onself to, rather than avoiding, the object or situation that is consciously or unconsciously feared.

countertransference The therapist's emotional reactions to the patient that are based on the therapist's unconscious needs and conflicts, as distinguished from his or her conscious responses to the patient's behavior. Countertransference may interfere with the therapist's ability to understand the patient and may adversely affect the therapeutic technique. Currently, there is emphasis on the positive aspects of countertransference and its use as a guide to a more empathic understanding of the patient.

cretinism A type of mental retardation and bodily malformation caused by severe, uncorrected thyroid deficiency in infancy and early childhood.

cri du chat A type of mental retardation. The name is derived from a catlike cry emitted by children with this disorder, which is caused by partial deletion of chromosome 5.

conversion symptom A loss of, or alteration in, voluntary motor or sensory functioning suggesting a neurological or general medical condition. Psychological factors are judged to be associated with the development of the symptom, and the symptom is not fully explained by a neurological or general medical condition or the direct effects of a substance. The symptom is not intentionally produced or feigned and is not culturally sanctioned.

culture-specific syndromes Forms of disturbed behavior specific to certain cultural systems that do not conform to western nosologic entities. Some commonly cited syndromes are the following: amok; koro; latah; piblokto; and windigo.

**D**

Da Costa's syndrome Neurocirculatory asthenia; "soldier's heart"; a functional disorder of the circulatory system that is usually a part of an anxiety state or secondary to hyperventilation.

decompensation The deterioration of existing defenses, leading to an exacerbation of pathological behavior.

defense mechanism Automatic psychological process that protects the individual against anxiety and from awareness of internal or external stressors or dangers. Defense mechanisms mediate the individual's reaction to emotional conflicts and to external stressors. Some defense mechanisms (e.g., projection, splitting, and acting out) are almost invariably maladaptive. Others, such as suppression and denial, may be either maladaptive or adaptive, depending on their severity, their inflexibility, and the context in which they occur.

déjà vu A paramnesia consisting of the sensation or illusion that one is seeing what one has seen before

delusion A false belief based on incorrect inference about external reality that is firmly sustained despite what almost everyone else believes and despite what constitutes incontrovertible and obvious proof or evidence to the contrary. The belief is not one ordinarily accepted by other members of the person's culture or subculture (e.g., it is not an article of religious faith). When a false belief involves a value judgment, it is regarded as a delusion only when the judgment is so extreme as to defy credibility. Delusional conviction occurs on a continuum and can sometimes be inferred from an individual's behavior. It is often difficult to distinguish between a delusion and an overvalued idea (in which case the individual has an unreasonable belief or idea but does not hold it as firmly as is the case with a delusion). Delusions are subdivided according to their content. Some of the more common types are: bizarre; delusional jealousy; grandiose; delusion of reference; persecutory; somatic; thought broadcasting; thought insertion.

delusional jealousy The delusion that one's sexual partner is unfaithful. erotomanic A delusion that another person, usually of higher status, is in love with the individual.

delusion of reference A delusion whose theme is that events, objects, or other persons in one's immediate environment have a particular and unusual significance. These delusions are usually of a negative or pejorative nature, but also may be grandiose in content. This differs from an idea of reference, in which the false belief is not as firmly held nor as fully organized into a true belief.

denial A defense mechanism where certain information is not accessed by the conscious mind. Denial is related to repression, a similar defense mechanism, but denial is more pronounced or intense. Denial involves some impairment of reality. Denial would be operating (as an example) if a cardiac patient who has been warned about the potential fatal outcome of engaging in heavy work, decides to start building a wall of heavy stones.

depersonalization An alteration in the perception or experience of the self so that one feels detached from, and as if one is an outside observer of, one's mental processes or body (e.g., feeling like one is in a dream).

derailment ("loosening of associations") A pattern of speech in which a person's ideas slip off one track onto another that is completely unrelated or only obliquely related. In moving from one sentence or clause to another, the person shifts the topic idiosyncratically from one frame of reference to another and things may be said in juxtaposition that lack a meaningful relationship. This disturbance occurs between clauses, in contrast to incoherence, in which the disturbance is within clauses. An occasional change of topic without warning or obvious connection does not constitute derailment.

derealization An alteration in the perception or experience of the external world so that it seems strange or unreal (e.g., people may seem unfamiliar or mechanical).

dereistic Mental activity that is not in accordance with reality, logic, or experience.

detachment A behavior pattern characterized by general aloofness in interpersonal contact; may include intellectualization, denial, and superficiality.

diplopia Double vision due to paralysis of the ocular muscles; seen in inhalant intoxication and other conditions affecting the oculomotor nerve.

disconnection syndrome Term coined by Norman Geschwind (1926¾1984) to describe the interruption of information transferred from one brain region to another.

disinhibition Freedom to act according to one's inner drives or feelings, with less regard for restraints imposed by cultural norms or one's superego; removal of an inhibitory, constraining, or limiting influence, as in the escape from higher cortical control in neurologic injury, or in uncontrolled firing of impulses, as when a drug interferes with the usual limiting or inhibiting action of GABA within the central nervous system.

disorientation Confusion about the time of day, date, or season (time), where one is (place), or who one is (person).

dysphoric mood An unpleasant mood, such as sadness, anxiety, or irritability.

displacement A defense mechanism, operating unconsciously, in which emotions, ideas, or wishes are transferred from their original object to a more acceptable substitute; often used to allay anxiety.

dissociation A disruption in the usually integrated functions of consciousness, memory, identity, or perception of the environment. The disturbance may be sudden or gradual, transient or chronic.

distractibility The inability to maintain attention, that is, the shifting from one area or topic to another with minimal provocation, or attention being drawn too frequently to unimportant or irrelevant external stimuli.

double bind Interaction in which one person demands a response to a message containing mutually contradictory signals, while the other person is unable either to comment on the incongruity or to escape from the situation.

drive Basic urge, instinct, motivation; a term used to avoid confusion with the more purely biological concept of instinct.

dyad A two-person relationship, such as the therapeutic relationship between doctor and patient in individual psychotherapy.

dysarthria Imperfect articulation of speech due to disturbances of muscular control or incoordination.

dysgeusia Perversion of the sense of taste.

dyskinesia Distortion of voluntary movements with involuntary muscular activity.

dyslexia Inability or difficulty in reading, including word-blindness and a tendency to reverse letters and words in reading and writing.

dyssomnia Primary disorders of sleep or wakefulness characterized by insomnia or hypersomnia as the major presenting symptom. Dyssomnias are disorders of the amount, quality, or timing of sleep.

dystonia Disordered tonicity of muscles.

**E**

echolalia The pathological, parrotlike, and apparently senseless repetition (echoing) of a word or phrase just spoken by another person. echolalia Parrot-like repetition of overheard words or fragments of speech.

echopraxia Repetition by imitation of the movements of another. The action is not a willed or voluntary one and has a semiautomatic and uncontrollable quality.

ego In psychoanalytic theory, one of the three major divisions in the model of the psychic apparatus, the others being the id and the superego. The ego represents the sum of certain mental mechanisms, such as perception and memory, and specific defense mechanisms. It serves to mediate between the demands of primitive instinctual drives (the id), of internalized parental and social prohibitions (the superego), and of reality. The compromises between these forces achieved by the ego tend to resolve intrapsychic conflict and serve an adaptive and executive function. Psychiatric usage of the term should not be confused with common usage, which connotes self-love or selfishness.

ego ideal The part of the personality that comprises the aims and goals for the self; usually refers to the conscious or unconscious emulation of significant figures with whom one has identified. The ego ideal emphasizes what one should be or do in contrast to what one should not be or not do.

ego-dystonic Referring to aspects of a person's behavior, thoughts, and attitudes that are viewed by the self as repugnant or inconsistent with the total personality.

eidetic image Unusually vivid and apparently exact mental image; may be a memory, fantasy, or dream.

elaboration An unconscious process consisting of expansion and embellishment of detail, especially with reference to a symbol or representation in a dream.

elevated mood An exaggerated feeling of well-being, or euphoria or elation. A person with elevated mood may describe feeling "high," "ecstatic," "on top of the world," or "up in the clouds."

engram A memory trace; a neurophysiological process that accounts for persistence of memory

epigenesis Originally from the Greek "epi" (on, upon, on top of) and "genesis" (origin); the theory that the embryo is not preformed in the ovum or the sperm, but that it develops gradually by the successive formation of new parts. The concept has been extended to other areas of medicine, with different shades of meaning. Some of the other meanings are as follows: 1. Any change in an organism that is due to outside influences rather than to genetically determined ones. 2. The occurrence of secondary symptoms as a result of disease. 3. Developmental factors, and specifically the gene-environment interactions, that contribute to development. 4. The appearance of new functions that are not predictable on the basis of knowledge of the part-processes that have been combined. 5. The appearance of specific features at each stage of development, such as the different goals and risks that Erikson described for the eight stages of human life (trust vs. mistrust, autonomy vs. doubt, etc.). The life cycle theory adheres to the epigenetic principle in that each stage of development is characterized by crises or challenges that must be satisfactorily resolved if development is to proceed normally.

ethnology A science that concerns itself with the division of human beings into races and their origin, distribution, relations, and characteristics.

euthymic Mood in the "normal" range, which implies the absence of depressed or elevated mood.

expansive mood Lack of restraint in expressing one's feelings, frequently with an overvaluation of one's significance or importance. irritable Easily annoyed and provoked to anger.

extinction The weakening of a reinforced operant response as a result of ceasing reinforcement. See also operant conditioning. Also, the elimination of a conditioned response by repeated presentations of a conditioned stimulus without the unconditioned stimulus. See also respondent conditioning.

extraversion A state in which attention and energies are largely directed outward from the self as opposed to inward toward the self, as in introversion.

**F**

fantasy An imagined sequence of events or mental images (e.g., daydreams) that serves to express unconscious conflicts, to gratify unconscious wishes, or to prepare for anticipated future events.

flashback A recurrence of a memory, feeling, or perceptual experience from the past.

flat affect An affect type that indicates the absence of signs of affective expression.

flight of ideas A nearly continuous flow of accelerated speech with abrupt changes from topic to topic that are usually based on understandable associations, distracting stimuli, or plays on words. When severe, speech may be disorganized and incoherent.

flooding (implosion) A behavior therapy procedure for phobias and other problems involving maladaptive anxiety, in which anxiety producers are presented in intense forms, either in imagination or in real life. The presentations, which act as desensitizers, are continued until the stimuli no longer produce disabling anxiety.

folie à deux A shared psychotic disorder between 2 people, usually people who are mutually dependent upon each other.

formal thought disorder An inexact term referring to a disturbance in the form of thinking rather than to abnormality of content. See blocking; loosening of associations; poverty of speech.

formication The tactile hallucination or illusion that insects are crawling on the body or under the skin.

fragmentation Separation into different parts, or preventing their integration, or detaching one or more parts from the rest. A fear of fragmentation of the personality, also known as disintegration anxiety, is often observed in patients whenever they are exposed to repetitions of earlier experiences that interfered with development of the self. This fear may be expressed as feelings of falling apart, as a loss of identity, or as a fear of impending loss of one's vitality and of psychological depletion.

free association In psychoanalytic therapy, spontaneous, uncensored verbalization by the patient of whatever comes to mind.

frotteurism One of the paraphilias, consisting of recurrent, intense sexual urges involving touching and rubbing against a nonconsenting person; common sites in which such activities take place are crowded trains, buses, and elevators. Fondling the victim may be part of the condition and is called toucherism.

fusion The union and integration of the instincts and drives so that they complement each other and help the organism to deal effectively with both internal needs and external demands.

# G

Gegenhalten "Active" resistance to passive movement of the extremities that does not appear to be under voluntary control.

globus hystericus The disturbing sensation of a lump in the throat.

glossolalia Gibberish-like speech or "speaking in tongues."

gender dysphoria A persistent aversion toward some or all of those physical characteristics or social roles that connote one's own biological sex.

gender identity A person's inner conviction of being male or female.

gender role Attitudes, patterns of behavior, and personality attributes defined by the culture in which the person lives as stereotypically "masculine" or "feminine" social roles.

grandiosity An inflated appraisal of one's worth, power, knowledge, importance, or identity. When extreme, grandiosity may be of delusional proportions.

grandiose delusion A delusion of inflated worth, power, knowledge, identity, or special relationship to a deity or famous person.

gustatory hallucination A hallucination involving the perception of taste (usually unpleasant).

# H

hallucination A sensory perception that has the compelling sense of reality of a true perception but that occurs without external stimulation of the relevant sensory organ. Hallucinations should be distinguished from illusions, in which an actual external stimulus is misperceived or misinterpreted. The person may or may not have insight into the fact that he or she is having a hallucination. One person with auditory hallucinations may recognize that he or she is having a false sensory experience, whereas another may be convinced that the source of the sensory experience has an independent physical reality. The term hallucination is not ordinarily applied to the false perceptions that occur during dreaming, while falling asleep (hypnagogic), or when awakening (hypnopompic). Transient hallucinatory experiences may occur in people without a mental disorder.

hedonism Pleasure-seeking behavior. Contrast with anhedonia.

5-HIAA (5-hydroxyindoleacetic acid) A major metabolite of serotonin, a biogenic amine found in the brain and other organs. Functional deficits of serotonin in the central nervous system have been implicated in certain types of major mood disorders, and particularly in suicide and impulsivity.

hippocampus Olfactory brain; a sea-horse¾shaped structure located within the brain that is an important part of the limbic system. The hippocampus is involved in some aspects of memory, in the control of the autonomic functions, and in emotional expression.

hyperacusis Inordinate sensitivity to sounds; it may be on an emotional or an organic basis.

hypersomnia Excessive sleepiness, as evidenced by prolonged nocturnal sleep, difficulty maintaining an alert awake state during the day, or undesired daytime sleep episodes. ideas of reference The feeling that casual incidents and external events have a particular and unusual meaning that is specific to the person. This is to be distinguished from a delusion of reference, in which there is a belief that is held with delusional conviction

hypnagogic Referring to the semiconscious state immediately preceding sleep; may include hallucinations that are of no pathological significance.

hypnopompic Referring to the state immediately preceding awakening; may include hallucinations that are of no pathological significance.

# I

id In Freudian theory, the part of the personality that is the unconscious source of unstructured desires and drives. See also ego; superego.

idealization A mental mechanism in which the person attributes exaggeratedly positive qualities to the self or others.

ideas of reference Incorrect interpretations of casual incidents and external events as having direct reference to oneself. May reach sufficient intensity to constitute delusions.

identification A defense mechanism, operating unconsciously, by which one patterns oneself after some other person. Identification plays a major role in the development of one's personality and specifically of the superego. To be differentiated from imitation or role modeling, which is a conscious process.

idiot savant A person with gross mental retardation who nonetheless is capable of performing certain remarkable feats in sharply circumscribed intellectual areas, such as calendar calculation or puzzle solving.

illusion A misperception or misinterpretation of a real external stimulus, such as hearing the rustling of leaves as the sound of voices. See also hallucination.

imprinting A term in ethology referring to a process similar to rapid learning or behavioral patterning that occurs at critical points in very early stages of animal development. The extent to which imprinting occurs in human development has not been established.

inappropriate affect An affect type that represents an unusual affective expression that does not match with the content of what is being said or thought.

incoherence Speech or thinking that is essentially incomprehensible to others because words or phrases are joined together without a logical or meaningful connection. This disturbance occurs within clauses, in contrast to derailment, in which the disturbance is between clauses. This has sometimes been referred to as "word salad" to convey the degree of linguistic disorganization. Mildly ungrammatical constructions or idiomatic usages characteristic of particular regional or cultural backgrounds, lack of education, or low intelligence should not be considered incoherence. The term is generally not applied when there is evidence that the disturbance in speech is due to an aphasia.

incorporation A primitive defense mechanism, operating unconsciously, in which the psychic representation of a person, or parts of the person, is figuratively ingested.

individuation A process of differentiation, the end result of which is development of the individual personality that is separate and distinct from all others.

indoleamine One of a group of biogenic amines (e.g., serotonin) that contains a five-membered, nitrogen-containing indole ring and an amine group within its chemical structure. inhibition Behavioral evidence of an unconscious defense against forbidden instinctual drives; may interfere with or restrict specific activities.

insomnia A subjective complaint of difficulty falling or staying asleep or poor sleep quality. Types of insomnia include:

initial insomnia Difficulty in falling asleep.

instinct An inborn drive. The primary human instincts include self-preservation, sexuality, and according to some proponents the death instinct, of which aggression is one manifestation.

integration The useful organization and incorporation of both new and old data, experience, and emotional capacities into the personality. Also refers to the organization and amalgamation of functions at various levels of psychosexual development.

intellectualization A mental mechanism in which the person engages in excessive abstract thinking to avoid confrontation with conflicts or disturbing feelings.

intersex condition A condition in which an individual shows intermingling, in various degrees, of the characteristics of each sex, including physical form, reproductive organs, and sexual behavior.

introspection Self-observation; examination of one's feelings, often as a result of psychotherapy.

introversion Preoccupation with oneself and accompanying reduction of interest in the outside world. Contrast to extraversion.

isolation A defense mechanism operating unconsciously central to obsessive-compulsive phenomena in which the affect is detached from an idea and rendered unconscious, leaving the conscious idea colorless and emotionally neutral.

**K**

Klinefelter's syndrome Chromosomal defect in males in which there is an extra X chromosome; manifestations may include underdeveloped testes, physical feminization, sterility, and mental retardation.

koro A culture specific syndrome of China involving fear of retraction of penis into abdomen with the belief that this will lead to death.

**L**

la belle indifférence Literally, "beautiful indifference." Seen in certain patients with conversion disorders who show an inappropriate lack of concern about their disabilities. labile Rapidly shifting (as applied to emotions); unstable.

labile affect An affect type that indicates abnormal sudden rapid shifts in affect.

latah A culture specific syndrome of Southeast Asia involving startle-induced disorganization, hypersuggestibility, automatic obedience, and echopraxia.

latent content The hidden (i.e., unconscious) meaning of thoughts or actions, especially in dreams or fantasies. In dreams, it is expressed in distorted, disguised, condensed, and symbolic form.

learned helplessness A condition in which a person attempts to establish and maintain contact with another by adopting a helpless, powerless stance.

lethologica Temporary inability to remember a proper noun or name.

libido The psychic drive or energy usually associated with the sexual instinct. (Sexual is used here in the broad sense to include pleasure and love-object seeking.)

locus coeruleus A small area in the brain stem containing norepinephrine neurons that is considered to be a key brain center for anxiety and fear.

long-term memory The final phase of memory in which information storage may last from hours to a lifetime.

loosening of associations A disturbance of thinking shown by speech in which ideas shift from one subject to another that is unrelated or minimally related to the first. Statements that lack a meaningful relationship may be juxtaposed, or speech may shift suddenly from one frame of reference to another. The speaker gives no indication of being aware of the disconnectedness, contradictions, or illogicality of speech.

## M

macropsia The visual perception that objects are larger than they actually are.

magical thinking A conviction that thinking equates with doing. Occurs in dreams in children, in primitive peoples, and in patients under a variety of conditions. Characterized by lack of realistic relationship between cause and effect.

manifest content The remembered content of a dream or fantasy, as contrasted with latent content, which is concealed and distorted.

masochism Pleasure derived from physical or psychological pain inflicted on oneself either by oneself or by others. It is called sexual masochism and classified as a paraphilia when it is consciously sought as a part of the sexual act or as a prerequisite to sexual gratification. It is the converse of sadism, although the two tend to coexist in the same person.

memory consolidation The physical and psychological changes that take place as the brain organizes and restructures information that may become a permanent part of memory.

mental retardation A major group of disorders of infancy, childhood, or adolescence characterized by intellectual functioning that is significantly below average (IQ of 70 or below), manifested before the age of 18 by impaired adaptive functioning (below expected performance for age in such areas as social or daily living skills, communication, and self-sufficiency). Different levels of severity are recognized: an IQ level of 50/55 to 70 is Mild;

an IQ level of 35/40 to 50/55 is Moderate; an IQ level of 20/25 to 35/40 is Severe; an IQ level below 20/25 is Profound.

MHPG (3-methoxy-4-hydroxyphenylglycol) A major metabolite of brain norepinephrine excreted in urine.

magical thinking The erroneous belief that one's thoughts, words, or actions will cause or prevent a specific outcome in some way that defies commonly understood laws of cause and effect. Magical thinking may be a part of normal child development.

micropsia The visual perception that objects are smaller than they actually are.

middle insomnia Awakening in the middle of the night followed by eventually falling back to sleep, but with difficulty.

mirroring 1) The empathic responsiveness of the parent to the developing child's grandiose-exhibitionistic needs. Parental expressions of delight in the child's activities signal that the child's wishes and experiences are accepted as legitimate. This teaches the child which of his or her potential qualities are most highly esteemed and valued. Mirroring validates the child as to who he or she is and affirms his or her worth. The process transforms archaic aims to realizable aims, and it determines in part the content of the self-assessing, self-monitoring functions and their relationships to the rest of the personality. The content of the superego is the residue of the mirroring experience. 2) A technique in psychodrama in which another person in the group plays the role of the patient, who watches the enactment as if gazing into a mirror. The first person may exaggerate one or more aspects of the patient's behavior. Following the portrayal, the patient is usually encouraged to comment on what he or she has observed.

mood A pervasive and sustained emotion that colors the perception of the world. Common examples of mood include depression, elation, anger, and anxiety. In contrast to affect, which refers to more fluctuating changes in emotional "weather," mood refers to a more pervasive and sustained emotional "climate." Types of mood include: dysphoric, elevated, euthymic, expansive, irritable.

mood-congruent psychotic features Delusions or hallucinations whose content is entirely consistent with the typical themes of a depressed or manic mood. If the mood is depressed, the content of the delusions or hallucinations would involve themes of personal inadequacy, guilt, disease, death, nihilism, or deserved punishment. The content of the delusion may include themes of persecution if these are based on self-derogatory~ concepts such as deserved punishment. If the mood is manic, the content of the delusions or hallucinations would involve themes of inflated worth, power, knowledge, or identity, or a special relationship to a deity or a famous person. The content of the delusion may include themes of persecution if these are based on concepts such as inflated worth or deserved punishment.

mood-incongruent psychotic features Delusions or hallucinations whose content is not consistent with the typical themes of a depressed or manic mood. In the case of depression, the delusions or hallucinations would not involve themes of personal inadequacy, guilt, disease, death, nihilism, or deserved punishment. In the case of mania, the delusions or hallucinations would not involve themes of inflated worth, power, knowledge, or identity, or a special relationship to a deity or a famous person. Examples of mood-incongruent psychotic features include persecutory delusions (without self-derogatory~ or grandiose content), thought insertion, thought broadcasting, and delusions of being controlled whose content has no apparent relationship to any of the themes listed above.

**N**

negative symptoms Most commonly refers to a group of symptoms characteristic of schizophrenia that include loss of fluency and spontaneity of verbal expression, impaired ability to focus or sustain attention on a particular task, difficulty in initiating or following through on tasks, impaired ability to experience pleasure to form emotional attachment to others, and blunted affect.

negativism Opposition or resistance, either covert or overt, to outside suggestions or advice. May be seen in schizophrenia.

neologism In psychiatry, a new word or condensed combination of several words coined by a person to express a highly complex idea not readily understood by others; seen in schizophrenia and organic mental disorders.

neurotic disorder A mental disorder in which the predominant disturbance is a distressing symptom or group of symptoms that one considers unacceptable and alien to one's personality. There is no marked loss of reality testing ; behavior does not actively violate gross social norms, although it may be quite disabling. The disturbance is relatively enduring or recurrent without treatment and is not limited to a mild transitory reaction to stress. There is no demonstrable organic etiology.

nihilistic delusion The delusion of nonexistence of the self or part of the self, or of some object in external reality.

nystagmus Involuntary rhythmic movements of the eyes that consist of small-amplitude~ rapid tremors in one direction and a larger, slower, recurrent sweep in the opposite direction. Nystagmus may be horizontal, vertical, or rotary.

**O**

object relations The emotional bonds between one person and another, as contrasted with interest in and love for the self; usually described in terms of capacity for loving and reacting appropriately to others. Melanie Klein is generally credited with founding the British object-relations school.

obsession Recurrent and persistent thought, impulse, or image experienced as intrusive and distressing. Recognized as being excessive and unreasonable even though it is the product of one's mind. This thought, impulse, or image cannot be expunged by logic or reasoning.

oedipal stage Overlapping some with the phallic stage, this phase (ages 4 to 6) represents a time of inevitable conflict between the child and parents. The child must desexualize the relationship to both parents in order to retain affectionate kinship with both of them. The process is accomplished by the internalization of the images of both parents, thereby giving more definite shape to the child's personality. With this internalization largely completed, the regulation of self-esteem and moral behavior comes from within.

Oedipus complex Attachment of the child to the parent of the opposite sex, accompanied by envious and aggressive feelings toward the parent of the same sex. These feelings are largely repressed (i.e., made unconscious) because of the fear of displeasure or punishment by the parent of the same sex. In its original use, the term applied only to the boy or man.

olfactory hallucination A hallucination involving the perception of odor, such as of burning rubber or decaying fish.

ontogenetic Pertaining to the development of the individual.

operant conditioning (instrumental conditioning) A process by which the results of the person's behavior determine whether the behavior is more or less likely to occur in the future.

oral stage The earliest of the stages of infantile psychosexual development, lasting from birth to 12 months or longer. Usually subdivided into two stages: the oral erotic, relating to the pleasurable experience of sucking; and the oral sadistic, associated with aggressive biting. Both oral eroticism and sadism continue into adult life in disguised and sublimated forms, such as the character traits of demandingness or pessimism. Oral conflict, as a general and pervasive influence, might underlie the psychological determinants of addictive disorders, depression, and some functional psychotic disorders.

orientation Awareness of one's self in relation to time, place, and person.

overcompensation A conscious or unconscious process in which a real or imagined physical or psychological deficit generates exaggerated correction. Concept introduced by Adler.

overdetermination The concept of multiple unconscious causes of an emotional reaction or symptom.

overvalued idea An unreasonable and sustained belief that is maintained with less than delusional intensity (i.e., the person is able to acknowledge the possibility that the belief may not be true). The belief is not one that is ordinarily accepted by other members of the person's culture or subculture

**P**

panic attacks Discrete periods of sudden onset of intense apprehension, fearfulness, or terror, often associated with feelings of impending doom. During these attacks there are symptoms such as shortness of breath or smothering sensations; palpitations, pounding heart, or accelerated heart rate; chest pain or discomfort; choking; and fear of going crazy or losing control. Panic attacks may be unexpected (uncued), in which the onset of the attack is not associated with a situational trigger and instead occurs "out of the blue"; situationally bound, in which the panic attack almost invariably occurs immediately on exposure to, or in anticipation of, a situational trigger ("cue"); and situationally predisposed, in which the panic attack is more likely to occur on exposure to a situational trigger but is not invariably associated with it.

paranoid ideation Ideation, of less than delusional proportions, involving suspiciousness or the belief that one is being harassed, persecuted, or unfairly treated.

parasomnia Abnormal behavior or physiological events occurring during sleep or sleep-wake transitions.

persecutory delusion  A delusion in which the central theme is that one (or someone to whom one is close) is being attacked, harassed, cheated, persecuted, or conspired against.

perseveration Tendency to emit the same verbal or motor response again and again to varied stimuli.

personality Enduring patterns of perceiving, relating to, and thinking about the environment and oneself. Personality traits are prominent aspects of personality that are exhibited in a wide range of important social and personal contexts. Only when personality traits are inflexible and maladaptive and cause either significant functional impairment or subjective distress do they constitute a Personality Disorder.

phallic stage The period, from about 21/2 to 6 years, during which sexual interest, curiosity, and pleasurable experience in boys center on the penis, and in girls, to a lesser extent, the clitoris.

phobia A persistent, irrational fear of a specific object, activity, or situation (the phobic stimulus) that results in a compelling desire to avoid it. This often leads either to avoidance of the phobic stimulus or to enduring it with dread.

piblokto  A culture specific syndrome of Eskimos involving attacks of screaming, crying, and running naked through the snow

preconscious Thoughts that are not in immediate awareness but that can be recalled by conscious effort.

pregenital In psychoanalysis, refers to the period of early childhood before the genitals have begun to exert the predominant influence in the organization or patterning of sexual behavior. Oral and anal influences predominate during this period.

pressured speech Speech that is increased in amount, accelerated, and difficult or impossible to interrupt. Usually it is also loud and emphatic. Frequently the person talks without any social stimulation and may continue to talk even though no one is listening.

prevalence Frequency of a disorder, used particularly in epidemiology to denote the total number of cases existing within a unit of population at a given time or over a specified period.

primary gain The relief from emotional conflict and the freedom from anxiety achieved by a defense mechanism. Contrast with secondary gain.

primary process In psychoanalytic theory, the generally unorganized mental activity characteristic of the unconscious. This activity is marked by the free discharge of energy and excitation without regard to the demands of environment, reality, or logic.

prodrome An early or premonitory sign or symptom of a disorder

projection A defense mechanism, operating unconsciously, in which what is emotionally unacceptable in the self is unconsciously rejected and attributed (projected) to others.

projective identification A term introduced by Melanie Klein to refer to the unconscious process of projection of one or more parts of the self or of the internal object into another person (such as the mother). What is projected may be an intolerable, painful, or dangerous part of the self or object (the bad object). It may also be a valued aspect of the self or object (the good object) that is projected into the other person for safekeeping. The other person is changed by the projection and is dealt with as though he or she is in fact characterized by the aspects of the self that have been projected.

projective tests Psychological diagnostic tests in which the test material is unstructured so that any response will reflect a projection of some aspect of the subject's underlying personality and psychopathology

prosopagnosia Inability to recognize familiar faces that is not explained by defective visual acuity or reduced consciousness or alertness.

pseudocyesis Included in DSM-IV as one of the somatoform disorders. It is characterized by a false belief of being pregnant and by the occurrence of signs of being pregnant, such as abdominal enlargement, breast engorgement, and labor pains.

pseudodementia A syndrome in which dementia is mimicked or caricatured by a functional psychiatric illness. Symptoms and response of mental status examination questions are similar to those found in verified cases of dementia. In pseudodementia, the chief diagnosis to be considered in the differential is depression in an older person vs. cognitive deterioration on the basis of organic brain disease.

psychomotor agitation Excessive motor activity associated with a feeling of inner tension. When severe, agitation may involve shouting and loud complaining. The activity is usually nonproductive and repetitious, and consists of such behavior as pacing, wringing of hands, and inability to sit still.

psychomotor retardation Visible generalized slowing of movements and speech.

psychosexual development A series of stages from infancy to adulthood, relatively fixed in time, determined by the interaction between a person's biological drives and the environment. With resolution of this interaction, a balanced, reality-oriented development takes place; with disturbance, fixation and conflict ensue. This disturbance may remain latent or give rise to characterological or behavioral disorders.

psychotic This term has historically received a number of different definitions, none of which has achieved universal acceptance. The narrowest definition of psychotic is restricted to delusions or prominent hallucinations, with the hallucinations occurring in the absence of insight into their pathological nature. A slightly less restrictive definition would also include prominent hallucinations that the individual realizes are hallucinatory experiences. Broader still is a definition that also includes other positive symptoms of Schizophrenia (i.e., disorganized speech, grossly disorganized or catatonic behavior). Unlike these definitions based on symptoms, the definition used in DSM-II and ICD-9 was probably far too inclusive and focused on the severity of functional impairment, so that a mental disorder was termed psychotic if it resulted in "impairment that grossly interferes with the capacity to meet ordinary demands of life." Finally, the term has been defined conceptually as a loss of ego boundaries or a gross impairment in reality testing. Based on their characteristic features, the different disorders in DSM-IV emphasize different aspects of the various definitions of psychotic.

psychotropic medication Medication that affects thought processes or feeling states.

**R**

rationalization A defense mechanism, operating unconsciously, in which an individual attempts to justify or make consciously tolerable by plausible means, feelings or behavior that otherwise would be intolerable. Not to be confused with conscious evasion or dissimulation. See also projection.

reaction formation A defense mechanism, operating unconsciously, in which a person adopts affects, ideas, and behaviors that are the opposites of impulses harbored either consciously or unconsciously. For example, excessive moral zeal may be a reaction to strong but repressed asocial impulses.

reality principle In psychoanalytic theory, the concept that the pleasure principle, which represents the claims of instinctual wishes, is normally modified by the demands and requirements of the external world. In fact, the reality principle may still work on behalf of the pleasure principle but reflects compromises and allows for the postponement of gratification to a more appropriate time. The reality principle usually becomes more prominent in the course of development but may be weak in certain psychiatric illnesses and undergo strengthening during treatment. reality testing The ability to evaluate the external world objectively and to differentiate adequately between it and the internal world. Falsification of reality, as with massive denial or projection, indicates a severe disturbance of ego functioning and/or of the perceptual and memory processes upon which it is partly based.

reciprocal inhibition In behavior therapy, the hypothesis that if anxiety-provoking stimuli occur simultaneously with the inhibition of anxiety (e.g., relaxation), the bond between those stimuli and the anxiety will be weakened.

regression Partial or symbolic return to earlier patterns of reacting or thinking. Manifested in a wide variety of circumstances such as normal sleep, play, physical illness, and in many mental disorders.

reinforcement The strengthening of a response by reward or avoidance of punishment. This process is central in operant conditioning.

repetition compulsion In psychoanalytic theory, the impulse to reenact earlier emotional experiences. Considered by Freud to be more fundamental than the pleasure principle. Defined by Jones in the following way: "The blind impulse to repeat earlier experiences and situations quite irrespective of any advantage that doing so might bring from a pleasure-pain point of view."

repression A defense mechanism, operating unconsciously, that banishes unacceptable ideas, fantasies, affects, or impulses from consciousness or that keeps out of consciousness what has never been conscious. Although not subject to voluntary recall, the repressed material may emerge in disguised form. Often confused with the conscious mechanism of suppression. resistance One's conscious or unconscious psychological defense against bringing repressed (unconscious) thoughts into conscious awareness.

respondent conditioning (classical conditioning, Pavlovian conditioning) Elicitation of a response by a stimulus that normally does not elicit that response. The response is one that is mediated primarily by the autonomic nervous system (such as salivation or a change in heart rate). A previously neutral stimulus is repeatedly presented just before an unconditioned stimulus that normally elicits that response. When the response subsequently occurs in the presence of the previously neutral stimulus, it is called a conditioned response, and the previously neutral stimulus, a conditioned stimulus.

residual phase The phase of an illness that occurs after remission of the florid symptoms or the full syndrome.

## S

screen memory A consciously tolerable memory that serves as a cover for an associated memory that would be emotionally painful if recalled.

secondary gain The external gain derived from any illness, such as personal attention and service, monetary gains, disability benefits, and release from unpleasant responsibilities. See also primary gain.

secondary process In psychoanalytic theory, mental activity and thinking characteristic of the ego and influenced by the demands of the environment. Characterized by organization, systematization, intellectualization, and similar processes leading to logical thought and action in adult life. See also primary process; reality principle.

sensory extinction Failure to report sensory stimuli from one region if another region is stimulated simultaneously, even though when the region in question is stimulated by itself, the stimulus is correctly reported.

separation anxiety disorder A disorder with onset before the age of 18 consisting of inappropriate anxiety concerning separation from home or from persons to whom the child is attached. Among the symptoms that may be seen are unrealistic concern about harm befalling or loss of major attachment figures; refusal to go to school (school phobia) in order to stay at home and maintain contact with this figure; refusal to go to sleep unless close to this person; clinging; nightmares about the theme of separation; and development of physical symptoms or mood changes (apathy, depression) when separation occurs or is anticipated.

separation-individuation Psychological awareness of one's separateness, described by Margaret Mahler as a phase in the mother-child relationship that follows the symbiotic stage. In the separation-individuation stage, the child begins to perceive himself or herself as distinct from the mother and develops a sense of individual identity and an image of the self as object. Mahler described four subphases of the process: differentiation, practicing, rapprochement (i.e., active approach toward the mother, replacing the relative obliviousness to her that prevailed during the practicing period), and separation-individuation proper (i.e., awareness of discrete identity, separateness, and individuality).

sex A person's biological status as male, female, or uncertain. Depending on the circumstances, this determination may be based on the appearance of the external genitalia or on karyotyping.

sign An objective manifestation of a pathological condition. Signs are observed by the examiner rather than reported by the affected individual.

shaping Reinforcement of responses in the patient's repertoire that increasingly approximate sought-after behavior.

sick role An identity adopted by an individual as a "patient" that specifies a set of expected behaviors, usually dependent.

signal anxiety An ego mechanism that results in activation of defensive operations to protect the ego from being overwhelmed by an excess of excitement. The anxiety reaction that was originally experienced in a traumatic situation is reproduced in an attenuated form, allowing defenses to be mobilized before the current threat does, in fact, become overwhelming.

simultanagnosia Inability to comprehend more than one element of a visual scene at the same time or to integrate the parts into a whole

sleep terror disorder One of the parasomnias, characterized by panic and confusion when abruptly awakening from sleep. This usually begins with a scream and is accompanied by intense anxiety. The person is often confused and disoriented after awakening. No detailed dream is recalled, and there is amnesia for the episode. Sleep terrors typically occur during the first third of the major sleep episode.

social adaptation The ability to live and express oneself according to society's restrictions and cultural demands.

somatic delusion A delusion whose main content pertains to the appearance or functioning of one's body.

somatic hallucination A hallucination involving the perception of a physical experience localized within the body (such as a feeling of electricity). A somatic hallucination is to be distinguished from physical sensations arising from an as-yet undiagnosed general medical condition, from hypochondriacal preoccupation with normal physical sensations, and from a tactile hallucination.

spatial agnosia Inability to recognize spatial relations; disordered spatial orientation.

splitting A mental mechanism in which the self or others are reviewed as all good or all bad, with failure to integrate the positive and negative qualities of self and others into cohesive images. Often the person alternately idealizes and devalues the same person.

stereotyped movements Repetitive, seemingly driven, and nonfunctional motor behavior (e.g., hand shaking or waving, body rocking, head banging, mouthing of objects, self-biting, picking at skin or body orifices, hitting one's own body).

Stockholm syndrome A kidnapping or terrorist hostage identifies with and has sympathy for his or her captors on whom he or she is dependent for survival.

stressor Any life event or life change that may be associated temporally (and perhaps causally) with the onset, occurrence, or exacerbation of a mental disorder.

structural theory Freud's model of the mental apparatus composed of id, ego, and superego.

stupor A state of unresponsiveness with immobility and mutism

sublimation A defense mechanism, operating unconsciously, by which instinctual drives, consciously unacceptable, are diverted into personally and socially acceptable channels.

substitution A defense mechanism, operating unconsciously, by which an unattainable or unacceptable goal, emotion, or object is replaced by one that is more attainable or acceptable.

suggestibility Uncritical compliance or acceptance of an idea, belief, or attribute.

suggestion The process of influencing a patient to accept an idea, belief, or attitude suggested by the therapist.

superego In psychoanalytic theory, that part of the personality structure associated with ethics, standards, and self-criticism. It is formed by identification with important and esteemed persons in early life, particularly parents. The supposed or actual wishes of these significant persons are taken over as part of the child's own standards to help form the conscience.

suppression The conscious effort to control and conceal unacceptable impulses, thoughts, feelings, or acts.

symbiosis A mutually reinforcing relationship between two persons who are dependent on each other; a normal characteristic of the relationship between the mother and infant child. See separation-individuation

symbolization A general mechanism in all human thinking by which some mental representation comes to stand for some other thing, class of things, or attribute of something. This mechanism underlies dream formation and some symptoms, such as conversion reactions, obsessions, and compulsions. The link between the latent meaning of the symptom and the symbol is usually

symptom A subjective manifestation of a pathological condition. Symptoms are reported by the affected individual rather than observed by the examiner.

syndrome A grouping of signs and symptoms, based on their frequent co-occurrence, that may suggest a common underlying pathogenesis, course, familial pattern, or treatment selection.

synesthesia A condition in which a sensory experience associated with one modality occurs when another modality is stimulated, for example, a sound produces the sensation of a particular color.

syntaxic mode The mode of perception that forms whole, logical, coherent pictures of reality that can be validated by others.

systematic desensitization A behavior therapy procedure widely used to modify behaviors associated with phobias. The procedure involves the construction of a hierarchy of anxiety-producing stimuli by the subject, and gradual presentation of the stimuli until they no longer produce anxiety.

**T**

tactile hallucination A hallucination involving the perception of being touched or of something being under one's skin. The most common tactile hallucinations are the sensation of electric shocks and formication (the sensation of something creeping or crawling on or under the skin).

tangentiality Replying to a question in an oblique or irrelevant way. Compare with circumstantiality.

temperament Constitutional predisposition to react in a particular way to stimuli.

terminal insomnia Awakening before one's usual waking time and being unable to return to sleep.

termination The act of ending or concluding. In psychotherapy, termination refers to the mutual agreement between patient and therapist to bring therapy to an end. The idea of termination often occurs to both, but usually it is the therapist who introduces the subject into the session as a possibility to be considered. In psychoanalytic treatment, the patient's reactions are worked through to completion before the treatment ends. The early termination that is characteristic of focal psychotherapy and other forms of brief psychotherapy often requires more extensive work with the feelings of loss and separation.

therapeutic community A term of British origin, now widely used, for a specially structured mental hospital milieu that encourages patients to function within the range of social norms.

therapeutic window A well-defined range of blood levels associated with optimal clinical response to antidepressant drugs, such as nortriptyline. Levels above or below that range are associated with a poor response.

thought broadcasting The delusion that one's thoughts are being broadcast out loud so that they can be perceived by others.

thought insertion The delusion that certain of one's thoughts are not one's own, but rather are inserted into one's mind.

tic An involuntary, sudden, rapid, recurrent, nonrhythmic, stereotyped motor movement or vocalization.

token economy A system involving the application of the principles and procedures of operant conditioning to the management of a social setting such as a ward, classroom, or halfway house. Tokens are given contingent on completion of specified activities and are exchangeable for goods or privileges desired by the patient.

tolerance A characteristic of substance dependence that may be shown by the need for markedly increased amounts of the substance to achieve intoxication or the desired effect, by markedly diminished effect with continued use of the same amount of the substance, or by adequate functioning despite doses or blood levels of the substance that would be expected to produce significant impairment in a casual user.

transference The unconscious assignment to others of feelings and attitudes that were originally associated with important figures (parents, siblings, etc.) in one's early life. The transference relationship follows the pattern of its prototype. The psychiatrist utilizes this phenomenon as a therapeutic tool to help the patient understand emotional problems and their origins. In the patient-physician relationship, the transference may be negative (hostile) or positive (affectionate). See also countertransference.

transitional object An object, other than the mother, selected by an infant between 4 and 18 months of age for self-soothing and anxiety-reduction. Examples are a "security blanket" or a toy that helps the infant go to sleep. The transitional object provides an opportunity to master external objects and promotes the differentiation of self from outer world.

transsexualism Severe gender dysphoria, coupled with a persistent desire for the physical characteristics and social roles that connote the opposite biological sex.

transvestism Sexual pleasure derived from dressing or masquerading in the clothing of the opposite sex, with the strong wish to appear as a member of the opposite sex. The sexual origins of transvestism may be unconscious.

trichotillomania The pulling out of one's own hair to the point that it is noticeable and causing significant distress or impairment.

## U

unconscious That part of the mind or mental functioning of which the content is only rarely subject to awareness. It is a repository for data that have never been conscious (primary repression) or that may have been conscious and are later repressed (secondary repression).

undoing A mental mechanism consisting of behavior that symbolically atones for, makes amends for, or reverses previous thoughts, feelings, or actions.

urophilia One of the paraphilias, characterized by marked distress over, or acting on, sexual urges that involve urine.

## V

verbigeration Stereotyped and seemingly meaningless repetition of words or sentences.

visual hallucination A hallucination involving sight, which may consist of formed images, such as of people, or of unformed images, such as flashes of light. Visual hallucinations should be distinguished from illusions, which are misperceptions of real external stimuli.

voyeurism Peeping; one of the paraphilias, characterized by marked distress over, or acting on, urges to observe unsuspecting people, usually strangers, who are naked or in the process of disrobing, or who are engaging in sexual activity.

## W

Wernicke's aphasia Loss of the ability to comprehend language coupled with production of inappropriate language.

windigo A culture specific syndrome of Canadians involving delusions of being possessed by a cannibal-istic monster (windigo), attacks of agitated depression, oral sadistic fears and impulses.

word salad A mixture of words and phrases that lack comprehensive meaning or logical coherence; commonly seen in schizophrenic states.

## Z

zeitgeist The general intellectual and cultural climate of taste characteristic of an era.

# BIBLIOGRAPHY

# BIBLIOGRAPHY

About Mental Illness, Major Depression, September 2006

Familydoctor.org, Depression: Electroconvulsive Therapy, April 2005

The American Journal of Psychiatry, Treatment of Primary Dysthymia With Group Cognitive Therapy and Pharmacotherapy: Clinical Symptoms and Functional Impairments, by Arun V. Ravindran, M.D., Ph.D., Hymie Anisman, Ph.D., Zul Merali, Ph.D., Yoland Charbonneau, M.D., John Telner, Ph.D., Robert J. Bialik, Ph.D., Andrew Wiens, M.D., Jack Ellis, M.D. and Jenna Griffiths, Ph.D., October 1999

British Medical Journal, Treatment for Chronic Depression: Cognitive Behavioral Analysis System of Psychotherapy. - Review - book review by Gary E. Myers, March 2001

Journal of Psychotherapy and Practice, Adding Group Psychotherapy to Medication Treatment in Dysthymia, A Randomized Prospective Pilot Study byDavid J. Hellerstein, M.D., Suzanne A. S. Little, Ph.D., Lisa Wallner Samstag, Ph.D., Sarai Batchelder, Ph.D., J. Christopher Muran, Ph.D., Michael Fedak, M.D., David Kreditor, M.D., Ph.D., 2001

American Family Physician, Depression in Women: Diagnostic and Treatment Considerations, July 1999

MayoClinic.com, Depression in women: Understanding the gender gap, September 2006

Mental Health America, Depression in Women, 2007

HealthyPlace.com, Depression in Women, 2006

About.com, Depression and Women, by Tracee Cornforth, February 2007

Cleveland Clinic, Depression in Men, 2005

Mental Health Association of Greater St. Louis, Depression - A Guide for Men, Date Unknown

National Institute Of mental Health, Men and Depression, 2005

Health Perspectives, Depression in Men, By Linda Richards, May 2004

UCLA Mood Disorders Research Program, Depression, 2006

# BIBLIOGRAPHY

Healthyplace.com, Depression Community, Causes of Depression, 2006

About.com: Depression, What Happens in the Brain That Causes Depression? by Nancy Schimelpfening, August 28, 2006

HELPGUIDE.org, Depression: Signs, Symptoms, Types, and Risk Factors, 2007

University of Michigan Depression Center, About depression, 2007

Irishhelath.com, Unlocking the causes of depression…,2007

HealthyPlace, Addictions Community, Co-Occurrence of Depression with Medical, Psychiatric, And Substance Abuse Disorders, 2000

Department of Psychiatry, Washington University St Louis, Depression Facts, December 2006

AllAboutDepression, Genetic Causes of Depression, September 2004

Better Health Channel, Depression and Exercise, June 2007

Holisticonline.com, Depression, Nutrition and Diet, 2007

American Psychiatric Association, Let's Talk Facts About Seasonal Affective Disorder (SAD), November 2006

Healthyplace.com, Depression Community, Types of Depression, 2006

National Alliance on Mental Illness, Seasonal Affective Disorder, 2007

British Medical Journal, Volume 295, Seasonal affective disorder: the miseries of long dark nights? Abas Melanie, Murphy Declan, December 1987

Mental Health America, Postpartum Disorders, August 2006

Medline Plus Medical Encyclopedia, Post-partum depression, January 2007

American Family Physician, C. Neill Epperson, M.D., Postpartum Major Depression: Detection and Treatment, April 1999

University of Michigan Depression Center, Major Depression Disorder, January 2006.

HealthyPlace.com, Depression Community, Major Depression (Clinical Depression), 2006

Psychology Information Online, Medication for Depression, Antidepressant Medications, 2003

PubMed, Family therapy and chronic depression.,(Abstract) by Keitner G.I., Archambault R, Ryan C.E., Miller I.W., August 2003

MentalHealth.com, Dysthymic Disorder, Treatment, by Phillip W. Long, M.D., August 1997

Healthline, Depressive Disorders, by Paula Ford-Martin, Teresa Odle, Thomson Gale, 2006

National Institute of Mental Health, Bipolar Disorder, January 2007

Psychology Information Online, Bipolar Depression, 2003

Medscape Today, Psychosocial Treatment of Bipolar Disorder, Interpersonal and Social Rhythm Therapy, 2003

Teen Depression, Causes of Teen Depression, 2005

HelpGuide.org, Teen Depression, A guide for parents and teachers, June 2007

Family First Aid, Teen Depression Statistics and Warning Signs, 2004

National Youth Violence Prevention Resource Center, Depression, 2002

WebMD, Depression Guide, December 2006

BBC.co.uk, Health, Conditions, Depression in elderly people, by Trisha Macnair, July 2006

The Doctor Will See You Now, Depression in the Elderly, by Rafi Kevorkian, M.D., May 2005

HelpGuide.org, Depression in Older Adults and the Elderly: Signs, Symptoms, Causes and Treatment, February 2005

National Alliance on Mental Illness, Depression in Older Persons, May 2003

Familydoctor.org, Depression in Women, September 2004

WebMD, Depression: Depression in Women, December 2006

# BIBLIOGRAPHY

## ABOUT THE AUTHOR

Dr Steven Thomas is a highly experienced and well regarded therapist, having produced a wide range of books and tutorials. His experience of working with depression, anxiety and bipolar related illnesses has been very successful and he has introduced many people to the 'multi-faceted' approach to therapy, believing that no single therapy is likely to be sufficient to produce good results in all cases. He is married with three children, and lives in the UK, where he works exhaustively in the field of mood therapy, including hosting a number of well-known and popular seminars.